ANTIHYPERTENSIVE DRUGS

Edited by **Hossein Babaei**

Antihypertensive Drugs
Edited by Hossein Babaei

Published by InTech
Janeza Trdine 9, 51000 Rijeka, Croatia

Publishing Process Manager Sandra Bakic

Technical Editor Teodora Smiljanic

Cover Designer InTech Design Team

Additional hard copies can be obtained from orders@intechopen.com

Antihypertensive Drugs, Edited by Hossein Babaei
p. cm.
ISBN 978-953-51-0462-9

Meet the editor

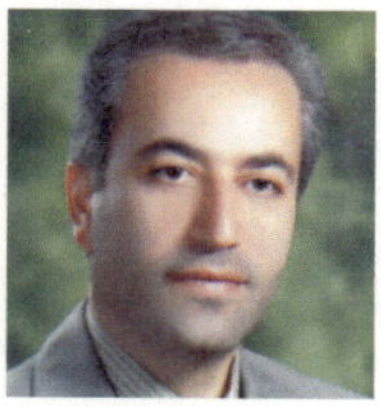

Professor Hossein Babaei obtained his Pharm D from Tabriz University of Medical Sciences in 1987 and his PhD in Cardiovascular Pharmacology from Bradford University (United Kingdom) in 1998. He is professor of pharmacology in School of Pharmacy, Tabriz University of Medical Sciences, Iran. He has been appointed as dean of Drug Applied Research Center, Tabriz University of Medical Sciences, in May 2003. Since then the research center has had greater academic achievements and according to Iranian Razi Research Festival, has been selected several times as top ranking among Iranian Biomedical Research Centers.

Contents

Preface

Hypertension or high blood pressure is widely prevalent and a major risk factor for cardiovascular diseases including coronary heart disease, myocardial infarction and stroke, and frequently causes damage to the arterial blood vessels, the eyes and kidneys. Prolonged hypertension can also lead to enlargement of the heart and may cause heart failure. This disease is usually asymptomatic until the damaging effects of hypertension are observed. Therefore, hypertension is known as the "silent killer." Several survey studies for assessing the burden of hypertension in different societies revealed that many subjects with hypertension were unaware of their disease, many of the aware subjects were not on treatment, and many of the treated patients were not controlled properly, particularly in developing countries. Hypertension afflicts more than one billion population worldwide and is a leading cause of morbidity and mortality. It has been predicted that in year 2025 it will increase by 24% in developed countries and 80% in developing countries. However, the expected increase may be much higher than these projections.

This book is another contribution to the application of new knowledge in the area of hypertension. Authors of this book are from different parts of the world sharing their new knowledge and experience in the direction of deep understanding and more clarification of the disease. They look from different angles to hypertension, providing an invaluable resource not only for clinicians, but also for all medical sciences students and health providers. I hope this book will provide new insight into hypertension disease and greater visibility and access to detection and treatment of vulnerable patients.

Prof. Hossein Babaei
Drug Applied Research Center,
School of Pharmacy,
Tabriz University of Medical Sciences,
Iran

1

New Therapeutics in Hypertension

Jorge Luis León Alvarez
Hospital Hermanos Ameijeiras,
Cuba

1. Introduction

Cardiovascular diseases are the leading cause of morbility and mortality worldwide. The main risk factor that contributes to the development of these cardiovascular diseases is hypertension. Hypertension increases the risk of injury in the vascular beds of various target organs such as retina, brain, heart and kidneys. Morbility and mortality associated with hypertension is associated mainly with cardiovascular complications. The main goal in the treatment of hypertension is not only controlling blood pressure (BP), but also reducing cardiovascular risk. (Chobanian et al., 2003)

The therapeutical management of hypertension has advanced considerably in recent decades, both in terms of its efficacy in available treatments as in its safety and tolerability profiles.(Table.1) Multiple effective antihypertensive drugs exist to carry out a logical choice. It is necessary to take into account the pathogenic alterations of renin secretion, sympathetic tone, renal sodium excretion, changes in cardiac output, peripheral vascular resistance and blood volume, without forgetting the individual considerations in each patient. However, none of the antihypertensive drugs currently available are able to control all cases of hypertension by themselves. For this reason, monotherapy alone is not usually able to lower BP to optimal levels in most patients. The use of combination therapy with antihypertensive drugs has become the norm. (Calhoun et al., 2008). However, the number of people with uncontrolled hypertension has increased, despite the innumerable evidence of the benefit of BP control and the advances in therapy. (Kearney et al., 2005)

At present the new knowledge obtained about the renin angiotensin aldosterone system (RAAS), the role of the endothelium and nitric oxide (NO), and the ion channels in the homeostasis of BP among others, have opened new lines of study. Therapeutical developments have recently emerged that could improve control of BP, either because they are new and alternative therapeutic strategies, such as carotid sinus stimulation devices, renal denervation and vaccination or due to the improved knowledge of existing alternatives.

This review will focus on little used antihypertensive drugs or on the emerging and application of new therapeutic strategies such as vaccination, renal denervation and the activation of baroreceptors.

2. Renin inhibitors

The importance of the RAAS in the pathogenesis of cardiovascular and renal diseases and hypertension among them has encouraged research to achieve blocking it partially or completely. The RAAS is composed of peptides and enzymes that lead to the synthesis of angiotensin (Ang) II, which effects are mediated by the action of AT1 and AT2 receptors and are involved in controlling cardiovascular function and hemodynamic equilibrium. (Morales Olivas & Estañ Yago, 2010)

After more than a century of research on the RAAS, Ondetti and colleagues, discovered in 1977 captopril (first inhibitor of angiotensin converting enzyme or ACE inhibitors). (Ondetti, Rubin & Cushman., 1977) In 1988, Timmermans and colleagues, (Timmermans et al., 1991) developed losartan (first AT1 antagonist receptor or ARBs). Both ACE inhibitors and ARBs have demonstrated their effectiveness in the control of hypertension delay, the natural progression of heart failure (HF), diabetes mellitus, and reverse target organ damage such as cardiac hypertrophy and thereby reduce cardiovascular and renal morbility and mortality. (Chobanian et al., 2003) It is not until 2007 that the Food and Drug Administration (FDA) approved the clinical use of aliskiren (first direct renin inhibitor taken orally). (Nussberger et al., 2002) This new group of drugs may represent a superior therapeutical strategy than that of other drugs that inhibit the RAAS, as they not only inhibit the actions mediated by Ang II synthesis but also the direct actions of prorenin and renin through the stimulation of prorenin receptors.

Decade	Antihypertensive drugs
1950	Reserpine, hydralazine, guanethidine, thiazide diuretics, ganglionic blockers
1960	Spironolactone, α 2 adrenergic receptor agonists, β blockers
1970	α 1 adrenergic receptor antagonists, ECA inhibitors, serotonin antagonists & agonists
1980	Calcium antagonists, imidazoline agonists, potassium channells openers
1990	ARBs, antagonist of endothelin receptors, aminopeptidase A inhibitors, crosslink breakers of the end products of advanced glycation, Rho kinase inhibitors
2000	Ouabain antagonists, urotensin II antagonists, vascular NAD(P)H oxidase inhibitors, modulators of the endocannabinoid, vasopeptidase inhibitors, renin inhibitors, vaccines, renal sympathetic denervation, Rheos system
2010	Dual inhibitors of neutral endopeptidase and angiotensin II blockers Dual inhibitors of endothelin converting enzyme and neutral endopeptidase NO releasing drugs with dual action: NO releasing sartans + NO releasing statins Dual antagonist of angiotensin II and endothelin A receptors

Table 1. Hystoric evolution in antihypertensive therapeutics.

Aliskiren is a potent non peptide renin inhibitor. When there is binding of aliskiren to the active site of renin (S1/S3), it blocks the activity of Asp32 and Asp215 of aspartate residue, thus preventing the conversion of angiotensinogen to Ang I. Aliskiren is a hydrophilic molecule with a high solubility in water, which facilitates their oral bioavailability. Aliskiren is absorbed via the gut, it has a bioavailability of 2.5 to 3%, but its high affinity for renin compensates the low bioavailability of the drug. Following oral administration, the peak concentration is reached within 3 to 4 hours. Its half life is 36 hours reaching its stable level in 7 days. Recent studies suggest that CYP3A4 is the enzyme responsible for aliskiren metabolism. 90% of aliskiren is purified through the feces. (Wood et al., 2003) In controlled clinical trials, aliskiren was shown to be as effective an antihypertensive drug as monotherapy or ACE inhibitors and ARBs. (Weir et al., 2007) Aliskiren is effective and safe in its combination with thiazide diuretics, ACE inhibitors, ARBs and blockers channels of calcium (Sica et al., 2006, Drummond et al., 2007, Andersen et al., 2008, Parving et al., 2008)

With respect to the incidence of adverse events, serious and non serious, there are no statistically significant differences between placebo and therapeutic doses of aliskiren, only at doses of 600 mg of the drug showed an increase in the number of patients who had diarrhea.

A comprehensive program of clinical trials: the ASPIRE HIGHER was assigned to evaluate the influence of aliskiren on cardiovascular and renal protection beyond their antihypertensive action. This big test covers four broad areas: the cardiorenal morbility and mortality, the cardioprotective, the renoprotective and hypertension with approximately 35,000 patients in 14 studies. (ASPIRE HIGHER Clinical Trial Program) the final results of three are already known.

In the study AVOID (Aliskiren in Evaluation of Proteinuria in Diabetes) aliskiren (150-300 mg/day) was administered to diabetic hypertensive patients with proteinuria. The study found that in 6 months of treatment, the addition of aliskiren to conventional therapy in patients with losartan 100 mg per day, conditioned a further reduction of 20% in the rate of urinary albumin excretion, with a reduction greater than or equal to 50% in the urinary excretion rate of albumin in 24.7% of patients receiving aliskiren compared with 12.5% of patients receiving losartan alone. An important aspect that is worth noting is that the rate of adverse effects did not increase in percentage or statistically with the addition of aliskiren to losartan therapy. (Parving et al., 2008)

The ALOFT study (Aliskiren Observation Of Heart Failure Treatment) evaluated the effect of adding aliskiren to the standard therapy for HF in a group of patients (including an ACE inhibitor or an ARBs, but not both, as well as betablockers and diuretics if needed). The addition of 150 mg of aliskiren conditioned significant reductions in natriuretic peptide (NP), proBNP, and echocardiographic parameters related to diastolic function of patients tested, compared with the group of patients who received conventional treatment. (McMurray et al., 2008)

In the study ALLAY (Aliskiren in Left Ventricular Assessment of Hypertrophy) a group of patients with hypertension, obesity and left ventricular hypertrophy were randomized to receive: aliskiren (300 mg), losartan (100 mg), or the combination of aliskiren and losartan with the doses mentioned. The primary endpoint was the evaluation of decreased left ventricular mass after 34 weeks of treatment in the groups already defined. Aliskiren provided a 15% decrease in left ventricular mass greater than the losartan, and the association of aliskiren and losartan provided a drop of 36% higher than losartan alone. This study confirmed the good tolerability of aliskiren and its combination with losartan. (Solomon et al., 2008)

Although the rest of the clinical trials that make up the ASPIRE HIGHER are not avaible, the use of aliskiren opens a new expectation, not only in the treatment and control of hypertension, but also due to its effects on target organ damage and the reduction of cardiovascular risk.

3. Imidazoline agonists

Many of the antihypertensive drugs that exert their action at the nervous system as methyldopa, clonidine, guanfacine and guanabenz, act by stimulating alpha 2 central receptors located in the pontomedular region and its effect consists in the reduction of the sympathetic outflow with a decrease in the peripheral sympathetic activity, but unfortunately they produce adverse reactions which include sedation, dry mouth and impotence, which high occurrence has determined a progressive decrease in their use.

In 1984, articles on imidazoline receptors located in the central nervous system are beginning to be published, and more recently, drugs capable of acting at this level leading to a peripheral sympathetic inhibition. This mechanism of action similar to the classic agonists differs mainly by a lower incidence of adverse reactions. (Yu & Frishman., 1996)

The existence of imidazoline receptors different from the alpha 2 was established in studies in the brains of cattle which tested the affinity of clonidine with these sites. However, because this drug shares its affinity for both imidazoline receptor as the alpha 2 receptor, new compounds were developed with high selectivity for imidazoline receptors, among which moxonidine and rilmenidine are of the most extensive development. Its action is performed on type I receptors, which include those that exert regulatory actions on BP. (Van Zwieten., 1996) There are also type II imidazoline receptors which are related to the stimulation of insulin release and some metabolic processes in the brain, but not involved in the regulation of BP. Type I receptors when stimulated with direct agonists such as moxonidine and rilmenidine, mediate a fall in BP and heart rate by peripheral sympathetic inhibition. The neural pathway involved has been suggested very similar to that dependent on alpha 2 adrenergic activation. (Chan & Head., 1996) In the case of moxonidine and rilmenidine, its action on type I receptors is predominantly exerted with minimal affinity for alpha 2 receptors.

The central action of the agonist of type I receptors has been demonstrated by studies in which stereotaxic injections have been used in parts of the central nervous system where vasomotor centers are located. The involvement of imidazoline receptors in the antihypertensive action of these compounds has been demonstrated with different techniques including antagonizing its effect through selective antagonists of these receptors. The antihypertensive activity occurs at the expense of reduced central sympathetic activity that leads to a reduction in peripheral vascular resistance and vasodilation. Stimulation of type I receptors by these agonists does not produce significant changes in cardiac output and heart rate, although suppression of episodes of tachycardia and antiarrhythmic activity has been reported. A reduction in plasma levels of catecholamines has also been shown. (Mitrovic et al., 1991)

In animal experimental models a reduction in the left ventricular hypertrophy has been shown, possibly due to sympathetic inhibition. Stimulation of type I receptors located in the kidney is involved to explain the natriuretic effect of these compounds. (Mitrovic et al., 1991) Oral administration of moxonidine determined maximum concentrations after 30 to 60 minutes. The absorption is higher than 90% and no first pass metabolism occurs in the liver. About half of the dose is eliminated without changes in the urine. Plasmatic half-life lasts about two hours but the antihypertensive action is much longer indicating an effect dependent on its accumulation in the central nervous system.

However, repeated doses are not accompanied by plasma accumulation. A glomerular filtration rate <30 ml/min should be considered a contraindication for use. The antihypertensive efficacy of moxonidine has been shown in controlled trials in which its effect has been compared with other classes of antihypertensive drugs that have included atenolol, hydrochlorothiazide, captopril and nifedipine. In all cases the effectiveness of BP control was statistically comparable. The antihypertensive effect is due to a vasodilator effect with reduced peripheral resistance without changes in heart rate and cardiac output. The administration of moxonidine produced a significant reduction in plasma catecholamine levels and long-term use determines reducing left ventricular hypertrophy without changing serum glucose and lipids levels.

The main advantage of moxonidine in relation to classical central agonists is given by a lower incidence of adverse reactions, even though there have been no studies comparing the two classes of drugs. Neither prospective studies have been conducted to demonstrate their protective effect on stroke, myocardial infarction, HF and kidney failure. The pharmacological characteristics of rilmenidine are very similar to those of moxonidine. Thus, experiments were made with a high number of patients in which its vasodilator effect as a result of reduced plasma concentrations of norepinephrine has been demonstrated. Another effect is the reduction of sympathetic baroreflex responses of heart and kidney, while vagal dependent cardiac baroreflex sensitivity is increased. As with moxonidine, left ventricular hypertrophy has proven reduction and be neutral on lipids and glucose levels. (Pillion et al., 1994)

4. Vasopeptidase inhibitors

In the early twenty first century vasopeptidase inhibitors were discovered as a new class of drugs for cardiovascular diseases by simultaneously inhibiting the angiotensin converting enzyme (ACE), thereby inhibiting the production of Ang such as Ang II, Ang 1-7 and Ang 2-8, completely blocking the substrates for the activation of AT1 and AT2 receptors and neutral endopeptidase (NEP), NEP metabolizes NP into inactived molecules, blocking this enzyme determines the increased blood concentrations of NP, such as brain NP, C and D, which decreases peripheral resistance and preload. It increases venous capacitance and promotes natriuretic action. There is a reduction in sympathetic tone, inhibition of catecholamine release and activation of vagal afferent endings, suppressing the tachycardia reflex and vasoconstriction, also promoting structural changes in the myocardial remodelling with a potent hypotensive effect. (Corti et al., 2001)

These drugs inhibit various metallopeptidases such as NEP, which catalyzes the breakdown of vasodilators and antiproliferative peptides (NP, kinins), ACE and endothelin 1. Several drugs of this group are known: omapatrilat fasidotril, mixampril, sampatrilat, CGS30440, MDL100, 240, Z13752A, among others. (Sagnella, 2002)

The most representative drug of this group is omapatrilat, a dual inhibitor of ACE and NEP. This inhibition results in an increase in vasodilator mediators (PN, adrenomedullin, kinins, prostacyclin-PGI 2, NO) and a reduction of vasoconstrictors (Ang II, sympathetic tone). Omapatrilat causes a reduction in systolic and diastolic BP higher than other antihypertensives (amlodipine, lisinopril), regardless of age, sex and race of the patient. It is well absorbed orally and reaches peak plasma concentrations of 0.5-2 h. It presents a half life of 14-19 h, allowing the administration of the drugs once a day. It is biotransformed into several inactive metabolites which are eliminated by the kidneys.

The OCTAVE study (Omapatrilat Cardiovascular Treatment Assessment Versus Enalapril) conducted in 25 267 hypertensive patients, confirmed the appearance of pictures of angioedema in omapatrilat treated patients, showing that the incidence of angioedema was 3 times higher than in patients treated with an ACE inhibitor, while in the OVERTURE (Omapatrilat Versus Enalapril Randomized Trial of Utility in Reducing Events) performed in 5770 patients with HF, functional class II-IV, ejection fraction ≤ 30% was 0.8% in patients treated with omapatrilat and 0.5% in those treated with enalapril. This dangerous side effect has stopped marketing the product. The simultaneous inhibition of ACE and NEP, both involved in the degradation of bradykinin, could lead to an accumulation of bradykinin and be responsible, at least in part, of the angioneurotic edema. (Sagnella, 2002)

5. Antagonists of endothelin receptors

Endothelins are a group of peptides discovered in 1988, produced by endothelial cells (ET-1, ET-2 and ET-3). They are one of the most potent vasoconstrictors known. The actions of endothelin ET-1 in humans are mediated through ETA receptors (present in smooth muscle cells of the vessels) and ETB (present on endothelial cells). Endothelins have been implicated in various cardiovascular diseases such as hypertension and HF. (Dhaun et al., 2008)

ET-1 acts on two receptor subtypes: the ETA, located in vascular smooth muscle cells, the myocardium, the fibroblasts, the kidney and the platelets, and the ETB, located on endothelial and vascular smooth muscle cells and in the macrophages. The ETA receptor stimulation produces vasoconstriction, fluid retention, proliferative effects, cardiac hypertrophy and releases norepinephrine and Ang II, and the ETB produces vasodilatation by releasing NO and eicosanoidsfrom endothelial cells and vasoconstriction by stimulating receptors on vascular smooth muscle cells. The ET-1, via ETA receptor stimulation also stimulates the release of cytokines and growth factors (vascular endothelial, of fibroblastic growth, platelet TGF-β) and facilitates platelet aggregation.

Several are the antagonists of endothelin receptors known so far as: ETA (darusentan sitasentan, LU135252); ETB (BQ788) and ETA/ETB (bosentan enrasertan, tezosentan). All these drugs produce beneficial hemodynamic effects in short term treatment, which raised great expectations in its use in hypertension treatment. There are numerous preclinical studies carried out in animals with antagonists of ETA receptors and ETA/ETB mixed antagonists, showing a decrease in BP in them.

Bosentan, a ETA/ETB mixed antagonist, has been used in clinical trials for the treatment of hypertension and HF, being effective in both situations and with tolerance generally acceptable in short term studies. Treatment with bosentan for 4 weeks reduced BP in hypertension as much as 20 mg of enalapril. It is important to notice that, this reduction was achieved without the activation of the sympathetic nervous system or RAAS.

In another study with darusentan, an ETA selective antagonist; in reducing systolic and diastolic BP compared with placebo was also effective. Its most common side effects are headache, facial redness and edema in lower extremities, and liver chemistry changes. Due to the limits of these studies, the role of these drugs is yet to be determined, because they have found significant adverse effects such as teratogenicity, hypertransaminemia and so its use has been limited by the FDA. (Krum et al., 1998)

The future of these drugs is uncertain. The results of human trials with these drugs have not reached the results from animal models. To date, these compounds have only been approved for use in patients with pulmonary arterial hypertension. Although they may reduce BP, there are antihypertensive drugs, safer and better tolerated available. However, the biological understanding of endothelin is rapidly evolving and its role in endothelial dysfunction of cardiovascular diseases is still a promising via in the pathogenesis and treatment of hypertension.

6. Ouabain antagonists

The sodium pump is the major cellular carrier system that controls sodium homeostasis and membrane potential, both key factors in the regulation of vascular tone and BP. Several experimental evidences suggest that increased endogenous levels of inhibitor prototype of the sodium pump, endogenous ouabain, may participate at least in part, in the pathogenesis of hypertension. (Hamlyn & Manunta., 2011) Chronic administration of ouabain to rats produces hypertension and increases, probably as a compensatory mechanism, negative endothelial modulation of vasoconstrictor responses produced by the endogenous vasodilator NO. (Manunta et al., 2009)

Endogenous ouabain is a fast action circulating hormone, which is present in several species. It is stored and secreted by the hypothalamus, the pituitary and the adrenal glands. In the latter it synthesized in the fasciculata cells zona from progesterone and pregnenolone through various isomers of 3β-hydroxyesters dehydrogenases. The synthesis in the hypothalamus and the pituitary gland has not been clarified yet. It has a half life of 5 to 8 minutes and is eliminated by the liver and kidney. It is humerally secreted by the exercise and the hypoxia through phenylephrine and Ang II by AT2 receptor by means of systems not yet well known. (Manunta et al., 2009)

On the other hand, for more than 200 years the ouabain (G-strophanthin) have been used to treat HF, an arrow poison of the African Ouabaio tree and of Strophanthus gratus plants. (Schoner.,2002). By radioimmunoassay techniques, it has proved that its half-life is of 21 hours in human and renal clearance. It has been found to be the predominant route of excretion and biliary excretion has been estimated at only 2-8%. (Selden, Smith & Findley, 1972)

The blocking action of cardiotonic steroids in sodium pump holds α receptors and has been shown in almost all animals and all types of cells. The sodium pump, the sodium (Na)-potassium (K) adenosine triphosphatase, Na+/K+-ATPase, has four isomers α receptors, α-1, α-2, α-3 and α-4. The α-1 is specific for Na+ and is present throughout the cell membrane. α-2 and α-3 receptors are less related to Na+ and are associated with the activity of the exchanger protein Na+/Ca^{2+}, NCX 1.3. Each cell type has a different proportion of these receptors, α-3 receptors are more numerous in nerve, myocardial and arterial smooth muscle cells, α-2 receptors are more abundant in striated muscle and α-1 receptors are more abundant in the kidney. The ouabain receptor acts mainly on α-3 and also in the α-2 recptors but with less affinity. Sperm has only the fourth receivers, the α-4 receptors. (Blaustein et al., 2009; Scheiner-Bobis & Schoner., 2008)

A new antihypertensive agent, rostafuroxin (PST2238) a digitalis derivative, has been developed due to the ability to correct abnormalities of the Na-K pump. It is endowed with high potency and efficacy in reducing BP and preventing organ hypertrophy in animal models. (Ferrari et al., 2006) At the molecular level in the kidney, rostafuroxin normalizes the increased activity of the Na-K pump induced by adducin mutants pump and endogenous ouabain. In the vasculature, it normalizes the increasement of myogenic tone caused by endogenous ouabain.

A very high safety factor is the lack of interaction with other mechanisms involved in the regulation of BP, along with evidence of high tolerability and efficacy in hypertensive patients point to the rostafuroxin as the first example of a new class of antihypertensive drug designed to antagonize endogenous ouabain and adducin. Phase II clinical trial was recently completed, Ouabain and Adducin for Specific Intervention on Sodium in Hypertension Trial (OASIS-HT), in which rostafuroxin was used with encouraging results as 23% had a significant decrease in BP. In the future we will have to wait to compare the results of rostafuroxin with other antihypertensive drugs to be validated as ACE inhibitors and ARBs and its influence on the control of BP. (Staessen et al., 2011)

7. Aminopeptidase A cerebral inhibitors

Aminopeptidases (AP) are proteolytic enzymes ubiquitously distributed, capable of hydrolyzing the aminoterminal amino acids of peptides and polypeptides that have an important role in controlling them centrally, as well as in peripheral tissues and blood. Their activities reflect the functional state of their endogenous substrates.

The terminology is confusing in relation to aminopeptidases, since the same enzyme is usually identified by different names. Aminopeptidase A (EC 3.4.11.7) hydrolyses the terminal of amino acids, mainly glutamic residues, but is also able to recognize the terminal of aspartic, so this enzyme is also known as aminopeptidase glutamate(GluAP).(Bodineau et al., 2008)

Several aminopeptidases (angiotensinase) are involved in the metabolism of the major active peptides of the RAAS. In particular, they are involved in the metabolism of Ang II, Ang III, Ang IV and Ang 2-10. Ang III is derived from the metabolism of Ang II by the action of the GluAP that hydrolyzes the peptide bond with an acid residue, Asp. The AlaAP and/or the ArgAP metabolizes Ang III to Ang IV by hydrolysis of the amino terminal Arg. The Ang I is transformed to Ang 2-10 by the action of the AspAP after the release of amino terminal Asp. The Ang III is a less potent vasoconstrictor than Ang II. It stimulates adrenal secretion of aldosterone, a neural stimulator and has the same affinity for the AT1 and AT2 receptors. Ang IV has little affinity for the AT1 and AT2 receptors and a lot for the AT4 receptor. Ang IV has an important role in regulating local blood flow, including the brain, but also has been assigned a role in cognitive processes, stress, anxiety and depression. Ang 2-10 opposes the vasoconstrictor effect of Ang II.

However, it is also said that this peptide would lead to aortic contraction dose dependent, through the AT1 receptor. Now, in regard to BP control, working with the hypothesis of a coordinated action of different peptides of the system acting together on the AT1, AT2 and AT4 receptors. Wright and colleagues (Wright & Harding, 1992, Wright & Harding, 1994, Wright & Harding, 1997) analysed the role of brain aminopeptidases in hypertension in several studies. They demonstrated that after intracerebroventricular injection of Ang II and

Ang III more sensitivity and a more prolonged increase in BP was observed in genetically hypertensive rats (GHR) than in normotensive Wistar-Kyoto (WKY) and Sprague-Dawley rats. But if previously treated with bestatin (an inhibitor of AlaAP and ArgAP), which prevents the conversion of Ang III to Ang IV, elevation of BP was enhanced and prolonged. These results indicate, therefore, that dysfunction in the central aminopeptidases activity could lead to Ang II and Ang III act longer and therefore, could carry out a progressive and sustained elevation of BP in RGH rats.

Later, Jensen and colleagues showed that in addition to bestatin, a GluAP inhibitor (amastatine), was injected by intracerebroventricular via, which inhibited the formation of Ang III, which is induced BP increase in rats WKYy the GHR so that there should be an effect mediated by the brain RAAS. They also noted that genetically hypertensive rats were more sensitive to the action of inhibitors than the normotensive ones. (Jensen et al., 1989)

RB150 is a prodrug with a specific inhibitory action on aminopeptidase A EC33, when administered intravenously, it inhibits cerebral aminopeptidase A, the Ang III formation and reduces BP over 24 hours in DOCA-salt rats. Thus aminopeptidase A cerebral inhibitors represent a potential antihypertensive treatment. (Bodineau et al., 2008)

In conclusion, although the discovery of ACE inhibitors and ARBs were two important milestones in the treatment of hypertension, the study of other RAAS components that act at both peripheral and central levels offer new therapeutic possibilities. The cerebral Ang III is a potent hypertensive factor. However, Ang 2-10 seems to contribute more to reduce hypertension. The results we have so far indicate that they fundamentally prevent the formation of cerebral Ang III, or perhaps also facilitates the formation of Ang 2-10, a line of research that could develop possible treatments for hypertension.

Therefore, recent studies on central inhibitors of GluAP, responsible for the formation of Ang III, may provide promising results. It is also increasingly clear that to properly understand the brain's control of the BP, studies should consider the bilaterally of the peripheral and central nervous system. The development of agonists and antagonists specific of the ACE-2, may offer an understanding of the pathophysiological role of ACE 2 in the modulation of the BP.

8. Modulators of the endocannabinoid system

The endocannabinoid system (ECS) is a new regulatory system capable of modulating a variety of physiological effects, consisting of endogenous ligands, specific receptors and mechanisms of synthesis and degradation. Endogenous ligands are a new class of lipid regulators among which there are amides and esters of polyunsaturated fatty acid chain. Endocannabinoids are defined as endogenous compounds, produced in different organs and tissues, capable of binding to cannabinoid receptors. The cannabinoids are synthesized "on demand", when they are needed, and released abroad immediately after their production. Its major molecular targets are the cannabinoid receptors (CB) type 1 and type 2 (Brown, 2007). The CB1 receptor is predominantly expressed in the central nervous system, but is also present at much lower, yet functionally relevant levels in various peripheral tissues, including the myocardium, postganglionic autonomic nerve terminals, and vascular endothelial and smooth muscle cells as well as the adipose tissue,liver, and skeletal muscle. The expression of CB2 receptors was thought to be limited to hematopoietic and immune cells, but they have recently been identified in the brain, the liver, the myocardium, and in the human coronary endothelial and smooth muscle cells. (Pacher et al., 2008)

Increased ECS activity also contributes to the generation of cardiovascular risk factors in obesity/metabolic syndrome and diabetes such as plasma lipid alterations, abdominal obesity, hepatic steatosis, and insulin and leptin resistance. However, the ECS may also be activated as a compensatory mechanism in various forms of hypertension where it counteracts not only the increase in SP, but also the inappropriately increased cardiac contractility through the activation of CB1 receptors. In addition, the activation of CB2 receptors in endothelial and inflammatory cells by endogenous or exogenous ligands was found to limit the endothelial inflammatory response, the chemotaxis, and the adhesion of inflammatory cells to the activated endothelium with the consequent release of various proinflammatory mediators, which are key processes in the initiation and progression of atherosclerosis and reperfusion injury as well as smooth muscle proliferation. (Pacher et al., 2008)

Currently, several types of endogenous cannabinoids have been identified, all of lipid nature and derived from polyunsaturated fatty acids of long chain. Anandamide (N-araquidonoiletanolamina, AEA) and 2-arachidonoylglycerol (2-AG) are the two best known endocannabinoids. AEA may be a partial or full agonist of CB1 receptors with low action over CB2 and 2-AG an agonist both of CB1 and CB2 receptors (Bisogno., 2008, Howlett., 2002).

The possible antihypertensive effect of cannabinoid ligands is based on the lowering of BP seen in the chronic use of cannabis in humans and in response to the acute or chronic administration of tetrahydrocannabinol in experimental animals. (Bisogno., 2008)

Recently there are results that demonstrate its high hypotensive efficiency in hypertensive animals compared with the normotensive ones and evidence that the tonic activation of the ECS in various experimental models of hypertension could be a possible compensatory mechanism. (Batkai et al., 2004, Wheal et al.,2007) This hipotensive tone could be attributed to a decrease in the mediated activity by the CB1 receptor in myocardial contractility rather than vascular resistance. So preventing the degradation of endogenous AEA by pharmacological inhibition of amidohydrolase fatty acid increases myocardial levels of AEA reducing BP and cardiac contractility in hypertensive rats but not in the normotensive ones. Perhaps the amidohydrolase fatty acid could be a therapeutic target in hypertension, where its inhibition would not only reduce BP but also prevent or stop the development of cardiac hypertrophy. (Lépicier et al.,2006)

The adverse side effects of these new drugs, their interaction with other ones, their pharmacokinetics, and their efficacy in the medium and long term, their probable use in other diseases are among the many questions that remain to be clarified in this new but promising group of antihypertensive drugs.

9. Urotensin II receptor antagonists

Human urotensin II (U-II) is a neuropeptide with the most potent vasoconstrictor action known to date. It is even 10 times more potent than endothelin 1. Although known since 1960, it only became a major goal of clinical research recently. It has a wide range of vasoactive properties according to their anatomical location and species studied.

The U-II binds to an urotensin II receptor, Gq protein (UT), originally known as orphan GPR14 receptor. This receptor has been identified in central nervous system cells, the bone marrow, the kidneys, the heart, the vascular smooth muscle and the endothelial cells. (Ames et al., 1999) Using immunohistochemistry techniques, U-II has been found in blood vessels of the the heart, the pancreas, the kidney, the placenta, the thyroid, the adrenal glands and in the umbilical cord. UT stimulation induces the release of NO, prostacyclin, prostaglandin E2 and endothelium derived factors that balance the contractile effect on vascular smooth muscle. Vasoconstriction is mediated by receptors in the vascular smooth muscle, whereas the vasodilatation is mediated by the endothelium. However, in HF and essential hypertension, the U-II loses its vasodilator capacity. So the U-II causes vasoconstriction of endothelium independently and vasodilatation of endothelium dependently.

The complex and contrasting vascular actions of U-II is not only dependent on the condition of the endothelium, but also on the type of vascular bed and species. (Ames et al., 1999, Liu et al.,1999, Matsushita et al.,2001, Maguire et al., 2004, Zhu et al.,2006)

In healthy individuals, the U-II acts as a chronic regulator of vascular tone. In patients with cardiovascular diseases, the balance is lost and elevated plasma levels of U-II in patients with HF, carotid atherosclerosis, kidney failure, diabetes mellitus, liver cirrhosis with portal hypertension and essential hypertension is found.

Endothelial dysfunction causes vasoconstriction or inadequate vasodilatation resulting in a myocardial ischemia and hypertension, associated with an increase in the U-II and UT. In fact, in patients with hypertension U-II is increased 3 or 4 times, and has shown positive correlation between HF and plasma levels of U-II. (Matsushita et al.,2001, Douglas et al.,2002, Richards et al.,2002, Cheung et al.,2004; Suguro et al.,2007)

Today there are several drugs that act on antagonism receptor of U-II: urantide, BIM-23 127, SB-611 812, palosuran. All at different stages of clinical research, so that in the coming years we will have results that allow us to evaluate the effectiveness on BP control and its impact on cardiovascular diseases. (Tsoukas, Kane & Giaid A., 2011)

10. Potassium channel openers

The openers of potassium channels (KCOs) are a class of drugs with an extreme chemical diversity; they include different structural classes such as benzopirans, cyanoguanidines, thioformamides, and pyrimidines. They base their action on the increase of transmembrane K^+ flow, resulting in a hyperpolarization of the cell membrane through the opening of potassium channels and the closing of Ca^{2+} channels, as a result the cell is less excitable and less prone to stimulation. There are two large families of potassium channels described in smooth muscle: channels regulated by voltage and channels regulated by ATP. (Moreau., et al. 2000) Potassium channels, regulated by intracellular ATP are located in the heart and blood vessels and are important modulators of cardiovascular function. The opening of potassium channels produces an increase in K^+ efflux from the cell so that the membrane potential at rest becomes more negative (hyperpolarization) and this leads to inhibition of calcium entry or an indirect antagonism of calcium, causing a drop in intracellular calcium concentration, relaxation of vascular smooth muscle cells and therefore vasodilatation.

(Wang, Long & Zhang., 2004) The primary target for KCOs action is through the regulatory subunit of the KATP channel, known as the sulfonylurea receptor or SUR, an ATP-binding cassette protein. (Moreau., et al. 2000)

These drugs came into use in 1980 in Japan with the commercialization of nicorandil, but now availability is wide and includes: celikalim, levcromakalim, birnakalirn, pinacidil, rilmakah, minoxidil, diazoxide and iptakalim among many others. KCOs like minoxidil, diazoxide, nicorandil, pinacidil, cromakalim and levcromakalim act by enhancing the ATPase activity of SUR1 subunit and the resultant channel opening causes hyperpolarization. (Sandhiya & Dkhar 2009)

Some of these drugs have been developed for clinical use and have several advantages such as its sustained and strong action on lowering blood lipids compared with other antihypertensive drugs.

The disadvantage is its lack of selectivity, thus besides smooth muscle cells, both the pancreas and the heart contain high concentrations of K^+ channels sensitive to ATP, so that the hypotensive effect is accompanied by other side effects such as hyperglycemia and cardiotoxicity, although changes in the chemical structure have produced good results, that are still not good for widespread use such as antihypertensive drugs. (Butera & Soll, 1994)

Diazoxide and minoxidil are currently recommended for the management of hypertensive emergencies and severe resistant hypertension, especially in patients with advanced renal disease. Their routine use as antihypertensive agents is limited because of a reflex increase in heart rate due to the stimulation of the sympathetic nervous system in response to arterial vasodilatation causing flushing, headache and/or sodium and water retention. Therefore, KCOs should be administered in conjunction with a diuretic and b-adrenergic blocker to control reflex increase in heart rate. An increase in plasma renin activity (largely due to activation of the sympathetic nervous system) and aldosterone level may also occur. Hyperglycemic effects of diazoxide and possible hypertrichosis with minoxidil also limit their longterm use, particularly in women. (Jahangir & Terzic 2005)

Recently a new KCOs sensitive to ATP has been developed: the iptakalim, which selectively relaxes small arteries with a more powerful action in hypertensive states. The iptakalim increases NO associated with increased intracellular calcium in cultured aortic endothelial cells. In addition, the iptakalim inhibits the synthesis and release of endothelin 1 associated with reduced RNA messenger of ET 1 and of the ECE. It inhibits the over expression of molecular adhesion in aortic endothelial cells subjected to metabolic disturbance induced by low density lipoprotein, homocysteine, or hyperglycemia, so it can reduce vascular and cardiac remodeling and endothelial dysfunction. (Wang et al., 2007)

Therefore, the protective profile of iptakalim may not only be due to the controlling of BP but may also relate to its effects in the endothelium system. Iptakalim has a selective antihypertensive efficacy with steady and long-lasting characteristics and produces less side and toxicity effects under the effective doses. It has the virtue for hypertension treatment by reversing hypertensive cardiovascular remodeling and protecting the target organs. (Wang, Long & Zhang.,2005)

However, cardioprotective and antiischemic properties of KCOs, beneficial effects on glycation and plasma lipids and bronchial smooth muscle relaxation still makes potassium channel openers an attractive antihypertensive class in patients with ischemic heart disease, diabetes mellitus and bronchospastic disease.

11. Vascular NAD(P)H oxidase inhibitors

The involvement of oxidative stress in hypertension is well known. There is strong evidence that oxidative stress is increased in essential hypertension, renovascular hypertension, preeclampsia and hypertension induced by cyclosporine.

Hypertensive patients have significantly higher levels of hydrogen peroxide (H_20_2) in plasma than the normotensive ones. Besides the normotensive ones which have a family history of hypertension have an increased production of H_20_2 than those who have no family history of hypertension, suggesting that there may be a genetic component in the high production of H_20_2. (Stocker & Keaney, 2004)

The NAD(P)H oxidase is the largest supplier of superoxide (O_2^-) in blood vessels and its expression and actions are regulated by Ang II through AT1 receptor. It has been shown that NAD(P)H oxidase contributes to the pathogenesis of hypertension. (Matsuno et al., 2005, Gavazzi et al., 2006)

The NAD(P)H oxidase is found in neutrophils and has five subunits: p67phox, p40phox, p22phox, and gp91phox catalytic subunit (also known as "NOX/DUOX family"), with 7 counterparts known to date, with diverse biological functions in different tissues such as: the colon, the blood vessels, the lungs, the heart, the kidneys, the nervous system, the ear, the bones, the testicles, the thyroid and lymphoid tissues. (S Wind et al., 2010)

Though the interaction of subunits in cardiovascular cells and its regulation and function of each NOX/DUOX is still uncertain, it is clear that NOX/DUOX enzymes are very important in normal biological response and contribute to cardiovascular and renal disease, including atherosclerosis and hypertension.

The development of specific inhibitors of these enzymes has attracted attention for its potential therapeutic use in hypertension. Experiments have shown that inhibitors of NAD(P)H decrease the release of O_2^- and increase the synthesis of NO, thus lowering BP. So far, two specific inhibitors: gp91ds-tat and apocynin have been proven to reduce BP in animals in labs. Other inhibitors such as diphenylene iodonium, aminoethyl benzenesulfono fluoride, S17834, PR39 and VAS2870, have proven to be effective in vitro, its effectiveness, pharmacokinetics and specificity is to be determined in vivo. (S Wind et al., 2010)

Many of these drugs not only inhibit the NAD(P)H oxidase but also other enzyme systems and cannot be administered orally, so its clinical use is limited. In addition, reactive oxygen species are so important to the immune and vascular health of human beings as for the disease, so not discriminating against the inhibition of NAD(P)H oxidase derived from reactive oxygen species could produce dangerous side effects.

Other drugs such as ACE inhibitors, ARBs and drugs lowering cholesterol like statins have also shown that they attenuate the activation of NAD(P)H oxidase, so this could be a promising avenue in the search for molecules with specific activities over enzymatic systems involved in cardiovascular diseases.

12. Vaccines

The first attempts to produce a vaccine for hypertension was conducted in the early 50s of the twentieth century and were focused on the RAAS. At that time immunogen renin was employed, demonstrating an antihypertensive action. However, its development was abandoned when observing the appearance of an autoimmune disease characterized by the deposition of antibodies antirenin in the juxtaglomerular apparatus and progressive interstitial inflammatory lesion in the kidney in animal models studied. (Goldblatt, Haas & Lamfrom, 1951, Michel et al., 1987)

Years later in the 60s, interest is focused on vaccines used against Ang I, but these had no antihypertensive effect. (Downham et al., 2003) At present, interest is focused on Ang II as an immunogen agent using a new immunization technology that combines antigens on the surface of a structure of virus like particles (VLP) generating a B cell response against autoantigens. VLPs conjugated to Ang II (CYT006-AngQb vaccine) have been tested in preclinical and clinical trials and have been observed to be well tolerated, immunogenic and with a high proportion of respondent individuals.

In Phase I studies, the tolerability, safety and immunogenicity of the vaccine was assessed after injection of the vaccine in 12 healthy subjects. They noted that the vaccine was well tolerated, safe and rapidly produced levels of specific antibodies to Ang II, which descended over time. (Ambühl et al., 2007) In Phase II B trials, in order to evaluate the effective response dose, the effect of the administration of 100 or 300 micrograms of the vaccine (CYT006-AngQb) or placebo to 72 patients (65 men and seven women with a average age 51.5 years) with moderate hypertension had been analyzed. The administration of the vaccine or placebo was performed at zero, four and twelve weeks. After twelve weeks of follow up, we observed that vaccination with CYT006-AngQb induced a dose dependent response, so that the title of antibodies to Ang II was greater in patients who received doses of 300 micrograms. The BP changes were evaluated at week 14. It was observed that patients who received 300 micrograms of vaccine significantly reduced the daytime systolic BP by 5.6 mmHg and diastolic by 2.8 mmHg compared with placebo recipients. (Tissot et al., 2008)

However, more studies on the beneficial effects of vaccination against hypertension are still needed, its long term effects, its influence on target organ damage and mortality.

13. Renal sympathetic denervation

The role of afferent renal nerves in the pathogenesis of hypertension has been well studied in animal models. Renal denervation in animal models with renal chronic or renovascular failure result in attenuation of the BP. The depressing effect of renal denervation in these models is not caused by changes in renin activity or sodium excretion, but with reduced adrenal sympathetic activity. These findings suggest that afferent renal nerves contribute to the pathogenesis of renovascular hypertension and renal failure, due to the increase of the sympathetic nervous system activity. Moreover, selective afferent renal denervation by dorsal rhizotomy has confirmed that the depressing effect of renal denervation in these models is due to the interruption of renal afferent activity. Similar reductions of muscle sympathetic nerve activity recorded in the peroneal nerve was observed after therapeutic nephrectomy in patients with advanced renal disease, confirming the relationship between afferent sensory fibers of the kidney and central sympathetic activity. (Fisher & Paton, 2011)

In a study coordinated by researchers at Monash University in Melbourne (Australia) and published in The Lancet, the use of renal denervation, a technique based on the use of a catheter to clear the neural activity of the kidneys, could be useful in the approach of people with resistant hypertension. The Symplicity HTN-2 trial was a multicenter, prospective, randomized, and controlled study about safety and efficacy of renal sympathetic denervation in patients with uncontrolled hypertension.

The device (Simplicity Catheter; Ardian Inc, Palo alto, California) is a catheter that is inserted through the end of the renal artery and then the tip is removed slowly, rotating and emitting radio frequency motions to suppress nerve activity. (Fig.1)

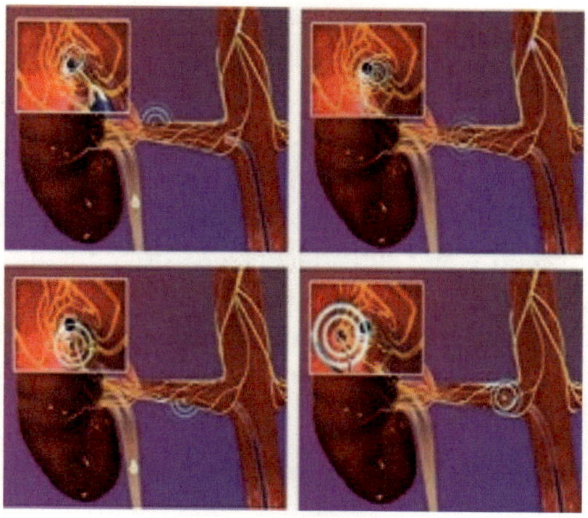

Fig. 1. Percutaneous renal denervation procedure. Graphic of catheter tip in distal renal artery. Reproduced from Krum, H. et al. (2009)

The study included a total of 106 patients from 24 hospitals in Australia and Europe. Both the treatment and control groups at baseline had high levels of BP (178/97 mmHg and 178/98 mmHg respectively), despite receiving intensive antihypertensive treatment, with an average of five drugs. After six months of beginning the trial, the average number of BP of the group that received renal denervation treatment was reduced to 146/85 mmHg, while the control group had a mean of 179/98 mmHg. (Krum et al., 2009)

Witkowski and colleagues evaluated the effects of renal denervation on BP and sleep apnea severity in patients with resistant hypertension and sleep apnea. They studied 10 patients with resistant hypertension and sleep apnea, who underwent renal denervation and completed 3 month and 6 month follow-up evaluations, including polysomnography and selected blood chemistries, and BP measurements. Antihypertensive regimens were not changed during the 6 months of follow up. Three and 6 months after the denervation, decreases systolic and diastolic BPs were observed. Significant decreases were also observed in plasma glucose concentration 2 hours after glucose administration and in hemoglobin A1C level at 6 months, as well as a decrease in apnea-hypopnea index at 6 months after renal denervation. (Witkowski et al., 2011)

In another study, a total of 11 patients received renal denervation treatment. Patients were followed up for 1 month after treatment. No periprocedural complications or adverse events during follow up were noted. A significant reduction of BP was seen at 1 month follow up.

Also, They noted a significant decrease in aldosterone level,while there was no decrease in plasma renin activity and in the renal function. (Voskuil et al.,2011)

Although the treatment is minimally invasive and presented no apparent complications, it is reserved only for patients with resistant hypertension unresponsive to adequate medical treatment. However randomized studies should be conducted with a larger population and a longer follow up term.

14. Baroreflex activation

The influence of the baroreflex in the control of the BP has been known for centuries. As long ago as 1799, Parry described for the first time in humans that carotid compression not only produced bradycardia but also hypotension. (Doumas, Guo & Papademetriou., 2009) When there is elevation in BP the baroreceptors are activated to decrease sympathetic outflow to the heart, kidneys, and peripheral arteries as well as it increases the parasympathetic tone in the heart. The result is a decrease in peripheral vascular resistance, heart rate and BP. The decrease in renal sympathetic tone reduces RAAS activity with resulting reduction of salt and water retention by the kidney and a decrease in the Ang II. The decrease in vasopressin arginine secretion observed during the increase in baroreceptor activity helps reduce systemic vasoconstriction and renal retention of water. That is why the regulatory role of arterial baroreceptors in the fluctuations of BP short term and sustained elevations in BP are well established. (Guyton et al., 1972)

On the other hand, there is accumulating evidence suggesting that sympathetic nerve activity plays an important role in the pathogenesis of essential hypertension. The findings indicate that sympathetic arousal is especially pronounced in patients who are difficult to control BP as in isolated systolic hypertension, hypertension associated with obesity and obstructive sleep apnea and in those with a non-dipper of BP pattern.

Early studies on the role of the baroreflex in the control of BP, were held in 1950 in dogs to which electrical stimulation of the carotid sinus was applied, showing significant decrease in BP in normotensive and hypertensive animals. (Morrissey, Brookes & Cooke., 1953) These data suggest that the baroreflex is important in chronic hypertension and renal sympathetic inhibition with an increase in natriuresis what could be the mechanism by which the baroreflex is involved in controlling long term BP.

After overcoming years of many technical difficulties, Tuckman implanted stimulators in both carotid sinuses allowing the regulation of stimulus achieving a BP reduction without adverse effects for a period of 2 to 18 months. (Tuckman et al., 1972) Other researchers conducted studies with similar results. (Parsonnet et al., 1969, Rothfeld et al., 1969, Brest, Wiener & Bachrach., 1972) Currently several studies are underway with a Rheos device that produces chronic electrical stimulation of the carotid sinuses (CVRx, MN, USA): European and U.S. study Feasibility and Rheos Pivotal trial. (Fig.2)

Rheos system includes a small pulse generator that is implanted under the collarbone, two thin wires that are implanted in the left and right carotid arteries and are connected to the pulse generator and Rheos programmer system: an external device used by physicians for non-invasive control of the energy delivered by the generator to the overhead wires. In the Device Based Therapy of Hypertension study (Debut-HT), 16 patients completed 2 years of follow up. Both systolic and diastolic BP decreased significantly with 35 ± 8 mmHg and 24 ± 6 mmHg, respectively. In 75% of patients, a decrease in BP of 20 mmHg in systolic BP was shown and 31% achieved BP control. (Scheffers et al., 2008)

In the European and North American study, Rheos system was applied to 16 patients with resistant hypertension which demonstrated a statistically significant decrease in BP in 3 months, along with reduction of left ventricular mass index (-24.1 ± 18.7 g/m^2), of the thickness of the septum (- 1.3 ± 1.8 mm), and of the thickness of the left ventricular posterior wall (-1.4 ± 1.1 mm). These results are also accompanied by reduction in the number of antihypertensive drugs used per patient. (de Leeuw et al., 2008) Another study of 12 patients with Rheos system in patients with resistant hypertension showed no deterioration of renal function after 1 year follow up. (Scheffers, Kroon & de Leeuw., 2008) In another 12 patients with resistant hypertension studied by Heusser, showed that electrical stimulation of the baroreceptors decreased systolic BP in 32 ± 10 mmHg, and this one correlated with a reduction in the muscle sympathetic nerve activity, the heart rate and the concentration of plasma renin. (Heusser et al., 2010)

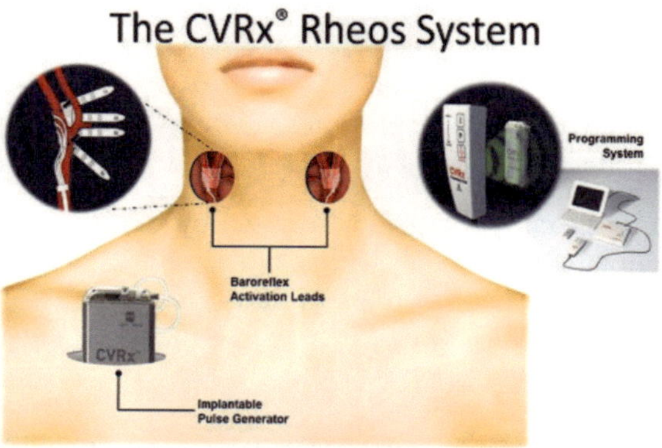

Fig. 2. Rheos System. From CVRx, Rheos, Baroreflex Hypertension Therapy are trademarks of CVRx, Inc. © CVRx, Inc. 2009

At the present time the company CVRx, Inc., the proprietress of this system has announced the introduction of a second generation with an implantable device: The Barostim neo™, with the characteristic to have a smaller generator and a 1 mm unilateral electrode, which should be utilized in resistant hypertension and the HF. (Hasenfuss, 2011)

Without misgivings another investigating step to explain details of efficacy to brief, middle and long term of these devices, their possible interactions with other drugs or surgical procedures, their medical indications, etc., what will permit in the future its use on a wider scale in the resistant hypertension.

15. Crosslink breakers of the end products of advanced glycation

The abnormal collagen cross links due to the formation of the end products of advanced glycation (AGEs) contribute to increase cardiovascular stiffness, which is a predictor of adverse cardiovascular events in old age, hypertension and diabetes. (Vlassara & Palace, 2002, Susic et al., 2004)

The first switch of the cross links of AGEs was phenacylthiazolium bromide (PTB), discovered in 1996, which reacts with cross links of AGEs derived from proteins. The PTB is rapidly degraded, so for the search of a more stable one, alagebrium (4.5 dimethylthiazolium or ALT-711) was discovered. (Dhar, Desai & Wu., 2010) Alagebrium breaks cross links of the end products of advanced glycation. In experimental animal models of advanced age, hypertensive or diabetic, the alagebrium reduced aortic stiffness and systolic BP, decreased the speed of pulse wave, improved diastolic ventricular compliance and cardiac output, improved diabetic nephrosclerosis and reduced urinary albumin excretion. Alagebrium also reduced oxidative stress in experimental elder animals by increasing the activity of glutathione peroxidase and superoxide dismutase. (Dhar, Desai & Wu., 2010) In elderly patients, alagebrium improved arterial compliance, reduced systolic BP and was well tolerated.

Today there are numerous studies underway in elderly patients with isolated systolic hypertension, HF and nephropathy; these results will clarify the likely benefit in the aging and cardiovascular diseases.

16. Rho kinase inhibitors

The intracellular signalling pathway of RhoA/Rho kinase (ROCK) is a mechanism discovered in the mid 90's of the twentieth century by japanese researchers, with a significant participation in the pathological remodeling of cardiovascular diseases. Two isoforms have been identified: the Rock 1 and ROCK 2. (Liao, Seto & Noma., 2007)

The vascular smooth muscle contraction is controlled by the concentration of free cytosolic Ca^{2+} and Ca^{2+} sensitivity of contractile proteins. The sensitization of Ca^{2+} in contractile proteins is determined by means of the RhoA/Rho kinase, which regulates the degree of phosphorylation of myosin light chains (MLC) by the phosphatase phosphorylation of the CLM, keeping the force of generation.

The contraction and relaxation of blood vessels is significantly regulated through phosphorylation and dephosphorylation reactions of the CLM in the regulatory subunit of protein phosphatase 1 target of myosin (myosin phosphatase target protein 1 or MYPT-1). It has been shown that the small GTPase Rho and its effector Rho A kinase modulate the phosphorylation of MYPT-1, so that when intracellular signalling pathway RhoA/Rho kinase is activated MYPT-1 increases. (Liao, Seto & Noma., 2007)

The route of the RhoA/Rho kinase is involved in pathological cardiovascular remodelling and in the regulation of BP and it is activated by agonists of receptors coupled to G membrane protein, such as Ang II, endothelin or noradrenaline, and produces contraction of the smooth muscle cells and hypertension. Rho kinase activation by Ang II is also involved in the oxidative stress and increased production of proinflammatory and profibrotic mediators. ROCK thus promotes oxidative stress and remodeling. (Liao, Seto & Noma., 2007)

Furthermore, RhoA-ROCK pathway is involved in cellular processes involved in the pathogenesis of various cardiovascular and renal diseases, as it participates in the effects of vasoactive and promoting of molecules of cardiovascular and renal remodeling, such as Ang II, 5 hydroxytryptamine, thrombin, platelet derived growth factor, endothelin, norepinephrine, thromboxane A_2 and U II. The activation of ROCK, a target of Rho A also produces a chain of cellular events such as the regulation of endothelial NO synthase expression by decreasing its gene activation of NAD(P)H oxidase with increased oxidative stress. (Liao, Seto & Noma., 2007) There is sustained evidence that Rho kinase pathway is substantially involved in the pathogenesis of vasospasm, atherosclerosis, hypertension, pulmonary hypertension, stroke and HF and increased central sympathetic nerve activity. (Rikitake & Liao JK., 2005)

The Rho kinase inhibitors (Y-27632, fasudil, hydroxyfasudil, KI-2309) induce relaxation of vascular smooth muscle, decrease in BP and inhibition of cardiovascular remodelling and endothelial dysfunction in hypertensive experimental animals. (Rikitake & Liao JK., 2005)

In hypertensive patients they improve endothelial dysfunction, normalize superoxide production, reduce peripheral vascular resistance and inhibit the development of cerebral and coronary vasospasm. (Masumoto et al., 2001) The first Rho kinase inhibitor approved for clinical use was the fasudil in 1995 in Japan and China, which has been used in cerebral vasospasm resulting from subarachnoid haemorrhage surgery. Several adverse effects such as intracranial bleeding, impaired liver function and hypotension have been reported. (Rikitake & Liao JK., 2005)

As more understanding of the physiological role of each ROCK isoform in the cardiovascular system is needed as well as the development of specific inhibitors of these to solve the specificity and safety of ROCK inhibitors.

17. Antihypertensive drugs with combined mechanisms of action

17.1 Dual inhibitors of neutral endopeptidase and angiotensin II receptors blockers

The Lancet in 2010 published the results of a study by Luis Ruilope and colleagues of LCZ696 a new drug (Novartis), which combines in a single molecule the double blocking action of Ang II and inhibits neprilysin (NEP 24.11) a metallopeptidase membrane that produces degradation of atrial natriuretic peptide, so it would provide the cardiovascular benefits of inhibiting RAAS without causing angioedema. (Ruilope et al., 2010)

This is a double blind multicenter study comparing the effects of LCZ696 with valsartan and another blocker of neprilysin called AHU377. It included 1 328 patients with mild to moderate hypertension, from 134 cities in 18 countries (Argentina, Canada, Denmark, Finland, France, Germany, Hungary, Italy, Latvia, Lithuania, Netherlands, Poland, Russia, Slovakia, Spain, Switzerland, Taiwan, and USA) who were treated between Oct/12/2007 and July/7/2008. Aged 18-75 years.

The patients were randomized to one of 8 groups of treatment: LCZ696 100 mg, 200 mg LCZ696; LCZ696 400 mg, 80 mg of valsartan, 160 mg of valsartan, 320 mg of valsartan, 200 mg AHU377, and placebo. The primary endpoint was the mean difference in diastolic blood pressure (DBP) compared among LCZ696 doses and valsartan doses (100 mg vs 80 mg, 200 mg vs 160 mg and 400 mg vs 320 mg) over a period of 8 weeks. The results showed that the decrease in DBP with the dual inhibitor is more effective when compared with valsartan, especially at 200 and 400 mg vs 160 LCZ696 and 320 mg of the latter. The DBP reduction with LCZ696 was a dependent dose. As data to highlight there were no significant adverse effects and no patients had angioedema.

Although, there were very promising results there is still much to clarify respecting its usefulness in the medium and long term, not only in the control of hypertension, but on the prevention and control of target organ damage.

17.2 Dual inhibitors of endothelin converting enzyme and neutral endopeptidase

Endothelin produced by endothelin converting enzyme (ECE) is a potent vasoconstrictor and profibrotic agent, while natriuretic peptides are degraded by NEP which have diuretic, vasodilator and antifibrotic properties, so that in a combination same drug of these actions could have a beneficial effect on cardiovascular remodelling, control of BP and cardiovascular mortality. Recently, several drugs have been synthesized: CGS 26303, CGS 34226, SLV88, SLV306 and SLV388, with which promising effects in experimental animals on cardiovascular hemodynamic independently of the BP have been shown. (Dhaun & Webb., 2011) That is why pre-clinical and clinical studies will be the future stage in these novel drugs.

17.3 NO releasing drugs with dual action: NO releasing sartans + NO releasing statins

Both hypertension and hypercholesterolemia are risk factors of cardiovascular diseases. Both produce endothelial dysfunction and promote the development of atherosclerosis. Increased Ang II levels are correlated with endothelial dysfunction and the expression of ACE activity is increased in hypercholesterolemia and atherosclerosis. Moreover, the oxidative stress is involved in many pathophysiological conditions in the cardiovascular system including hypercholesterolemia, hypertension, diabetes and HF.

The Ang II and the activation of AT1 receptors stimulate NAD(P)H oxidase, generating reactive oxygen species in vascular cells and thus endothelial dysfunction. It has been shown that NO is involved in modulating numerous vital functions and its role is known as the regulator of cardiovascular homeostasis, inflammatory response and cell proliferation of vascular smooth muscle.

The beneficial effects of inhibitors of hydroxy methylglutaryl CoA reductase 3 (statins) have been well tested in the treatment of hypercholesterolemia, a condition which is strongly associated with the development of atherosclerosis. In addition, statins significantly reduce cardiovascular mortality in patients with cardiovascular disease risk and which have direct effects on atherosclerotic plaque stability, NO metabolism, inflammation, endothelial function, oxidative stress and thrombosis. (Shepherd et al., 1995)

Moreover ARBs or sartans have demonstrated its safety and efficacy in controlling hypertension, they have reduced endothelial dysfunction and decreased cardiovascular morbility and mortality in diabetic patients, in hypertensive ones with HF and coronary artery disease. (Brenner et al.,2001, Cohn & Tognoni.,2001, Lewis et al.,2001, Dahlof et al.,2002, Pfeffer et al.,2003) Currently, there are drugs being developed that combine the antihypertensive action of ARBs with the releasing of NO in a single molecule, with the aim of improving the safety profile and effectiveness of their native drugs. Hybrids which combine the action of ARBs with a NO releasing statin, (also called statins sartans-NO), antagonize the effects of Ang II in experimental animals with similar power than losartan or captopril. (Nickenig, 2004) The nitric ester derivatives of pravastatin (NCX 6550) and fluvastatin (NCX 6553) have demonstrated antiinflammatory and antiproliferative action, so it has potential application in diseases with endothelial dysfunction and vascular inflammation. There are additional properties that make NO releasing statins more effective than the native ones. It has been shown that NCX 6550 inhibits platelet aggregation in vitro and reduces mortality in thromboembolism in experimental animals. (Dever et al., 2007)

Thus, the combination of the beneficial effect of ARBs and statins in a single drug may not only be favorable for the prevention of cardiovascular disease but also contribute to adherence of treatment in patients that need this therapeutics for a long period of time.

17.4 Dual antagonist of angiotensin II and endothelin A receptors

Known is the role of Ang II and ET1 in the pathogenesis of essential hypertension. These substances produce vasoconstriction through the activation of its receptors in vascular smooth muscle: the AT1 and ETA, respectively. Ang II promotes the production of endothelin and endothelin in turn increases the synthesis of Ang II.

Moreover, evidence suggests the interrelation between the endocrine and paracrine systems of Ang II and endothelin. Ang II increases the expression of RNA messenger in endothelial cells. Ang II stimulates the release of ET1 by endothelial cells involving AT1 receptors, Ca_2^+ mobilization and activation of kinase C protein. ARBs produce a significant decrease in BP and reduce endothelial dysfunction and cardiovascular mortality in hypertensive, diabetic and HF patients. Thus, the activation of ETA and/or ETB receptors of ET1 causes contraction of vascular smooth muscle cells and increases BP and an antagonist of ETA/ETB receptors like bosetan decreases BP in patients with essential hypertension. Thus the combination in one same drug of properties AT1/ETA receptors antagonists may have a greater effect than either drug alone and with fewer side effects. Today ETA receptor blockers have been modified to acquire AT1 receptor antagonism.

There are several compounds (MS-248 360, BMS-248360, SB-290 670) that in laboratory animals decreased BP, but these investigations are still in very early stages. (Kowal et al., 2004) But this new class of antihypertensive drug which simultaneously antagonizes the AT1 and ETA receptors promise to be a novel approach in the treatment of hypertension and other cardiovascular diseases.

18. Conclusions

The development of research at the dawn of the millennium, in nanotechnology, genetic engineering and biotechnology for the understanding of the multiple pathogenic mechanisms of cardiovascular diseases and its consequences and hypertension within them, have caused a real boom in the appearance of new therapeutic options for hypertension. About some of them (those that are the most in advanced stages of preclinical and clinical research) we have tried to give a small and modest updating.

Others in earlier stages of experimental research as antagonists of vasopressin receptors (RWJ-676070), NO stimulators and stabilizers: L-arginine, tetrahydrobiopterin (BH4), phosphodiesterase inhibitors PDE-5, N-acetylcysteine, donors of NO (NCX-899, naproxcinod, LA419), stimulators and activators of cyclic monophosphate guanosine (cGMP): BAY 41-2272, BAY 58-2667, BAY 41-8543, BAY 41-2272, HMR-1766, prostacyclin analogue (beraprost, ecraprost) thromboxane antagonists (KT2-962) and molecules with properties of triple inhibition ECA/ECE-1/EPN with CGS35601, yet there is little published data that permit a satisfactory evaluation. (Trapani et al., 2004, Battistini, Daull & Jeng., 2005)

However, what has been so far advanced allows us to have useful drugs with proven scientific evidence on cardiovascular risk reduction and augur a promising future in reducing cardiovascular morbility and mortality.

19. References

Ambühl, PM. et al. (2007). A vaccine for hypertension based on virus-like particles: preclinical efficacy and phase I safety and immunogenicity. *J Hypertens*, Vol. 25, No. 1 (Jan 2007), pp. 63-72, ISSN: 1473-5598

Ames, RS. et al. (1999). Human urotensin II is a potent vasoconstrictor and agonist for the orphan receptor GPR14. *Nature*, Vol. 401, No. 6750 (Sept 1999), pp. 282–286, ISSN: 0028-0836

Andersen, K. et al. (2008). Comparative efficacy and safety of aliskiren, an oral direct renin inhibitor, and ramipril in hypertension: a 6-month, randomized, double-blind trial. *J Hypertens,* Vol.26, No. 3, (Mar 2008), pp.589-99, ISSN: 1473-5598

ASPIRE HIGHER Clinical Trial Program. Novartis International AG 2008. Available from: http://www.novartis.com

Batkai, S. et al. 2004. Endocannabinoids acting at cannabinoid-1 receptors regulate cardiovascular function in hypertension. *Circulation,* Vol.110, No. 14, (Oct 2004), pp. 1996-2002, ISSN: 0009-7322

Battistini, B., Daull, P. & Jeng, AY. (2005). CGS 35601, a triple inhibitor of angiotensin converting enzyme, neutral endopeptidase and endothelin converting enzyme. *Cardiovasc Drug Rev*, Vol. 23, No. 4, (Winter 2005), pp. 317-30, ISSN: 1527-3466

Bisogno, T. (2008). Endogenous cannabinoids: Structure and metabolism. *J Neuroendocrinol,* Vol. 20, Suppl 1, (May 2008), pp. 1-9, ISSN: 1365-2826

Blaustein, MP. et al. (2009).The Pump, the Exchanger and Endogenous Ouabain: Signaling Mechanisms that Link Salt Retention to Hypertension. *Hypertension*, Vol.53, No.2, (Feb 2009), pp. 291–298, ISSN: 0194-911X

Bodineau, L. et al. (2008). Orally active aminopeptidase A inhibitors reduce blood pressure. A new strategy for treating hipertensión. *Hipertensión*, Vol.51, No.5, (May 2008), pp.1318-1325, ISSN: 1524-4563

Brenner, BM. et al. (2001). Effects of losartan on renal and cardiovascular outcomes in patients with type 2 diabetes and nephropathy. *N Engl J Med*, Vol. 345, No. 5, (May 2001), pp. 861–869, ISSN: 0028-4793

Brest, AN., Wiener, L. & Bachrach, B. (1972). Bilateral carotid sinus nerve stimulation in the treatment of hypertension. *Am J Cardiol,* Vol.29, No. 6, (Jun 1972), pp. 821-825, ISSN: 0002-9149

Brown, AJ. (2007). Novel cannabinoid receptors. *Br J Pharmacol*, Vol. 152, No.5, (Nov 2007), pp.567-75, ISSN: 1476-5381

Butera, JA. & Soll, RM. (1994). Recent advances in potassium channel openers: patent activity June 1992 to August 1993. *Exp. Opin. Ther. Patents*, Vol. 4, No.4, (Apr 1994), pp.395-408, ISSN: 1744-7674

Calhoun, DA. et al. (2008). Resistant hypertension: diagnosis, evaluation, and treatment. A Scientific Statement from the American Heart Association Professional Education Committee of the Council for High Blood Pressure Research. *Circulation*, Vol. 117, No. 25, (Jun 2008), pp. e 510-26, ISSN: 1524-4539

Chan, CK. & Head GA. (1996). Relative importance of central imidazoline receptors for the antihypertensive effects of moxonidine and rilmenidine. *J Hypertens*, Vol. 14, No.7, (Jul 1996), pp.855-864, ISSN: 1473-5598

Cheung, BMY. et al. (2004). Plasma concentration of urotensin II is raised in hypertension. *J. Hypertens*, Vol.22, No.7, (Jul 2004), pp.1341–1344, ISSN: 1473-5598

Chobanian, AV. et al. (2003). The Seventh Report of the Joint National Committee on Prevention, Detection, Evaluation, and Treatment of High Blood Pressure: the JNC 7 report. *JAMA*, Vol.289, No. 19, (May 2003), pp. 2560-2572, ISSN: 1538-3598

Cohn, JN. & Tognoni, G. (2001).A randomized trial of the angiotensin-receptor blocker valsartan in chronic heart failure. *N Engl J Med*, Vol. 345, No. 23, (Dec 2001), pp. 1667–1675, ISSN: 0028-4793

Corti, R. et al. (2001).Vasopeptidase Inhibitors: A New Therapeutic Concept in Cardiovascular Disease? *Circulation*, Vol. 104, No. 15, (Oct 2001), pp.1856-1862, ISSN: 1524-4539

Dahlof, B. et al. (2002). Cardiovascular morbidity and mortality in the Losartan Intervention For Endpoint reduction in hypertension study (LIFE): a randomised trial against atenolol. *Lancet*, Vol. 359, No. 9311, (Mar 2002), pp.995–1003, ISSN: 0140-6736

de Leeuw P, et al.(2008) Left ventricular reverse remodeling with chronic treatment of resistant hypertension using an implantable device: results from European and United States trials of the Rheos baroreflex hypertension therapy system. *J Hypertens*, Vol.26, Suppl 1, (2008), pp.S471, ISSN: 0952-1178

Dever, G. et al. (2007). The nitric oxide donating pravastatin derivative, NCX 6550[(1S[1alpha(betaS, delta S), 2alpha, 6alpha, 8beta-(R), 8a alpha]]-1,2,6,7,8,8a Hexahydrobeta,delta,6-trihydroxy-2-methyl-8 (2-methyl 1 oxobutoxy)1naphtalene heptanoic acid 4-(nitrooxy)butyl ester)], reduces splenocyte adhesion and reactive oxygen species generation in normal and atherosclerotic mice. *J Pharmacol Exp Ther*, Vol. 320, No. 1, (Jan 2007),pp. 419-26, ISSN: 1521-013

Dhar, A., Desai, KM. & Wu, L. (2010). Alagebrium attenuates acute methylglyoxal-induced glucose intolerance in Sprague-Dawley rats. *British Journal of Pharmacology*, Vol.159, No. 1, (Jan 2010), pp.166–175, ISSN: 1476-5381

Dhaun, N. & Webb, DJ. (2011). Dual Endothelin-Converting Enzyme/Neutral Endopeptidase Inhibition: A Novel Treatment for Renovascular Hypertension Beyond Blood Pressure Lowering? *Hypertension*, Vol.57, No. 4, (Apr 2011), pp.667-669, ISSN: 1524-4563

Dhaun, N. et al. (2008). Role of Endothelin-1 in Clinical Hypertension 20 Years On. *Hypertension*, Vol. 52, No. 3, (Sept 2008), pp.452-459, ISSN : 1524-4563

Douglas, SA. et al. (2000). Differential vasoconstrictor activity of human urotensin II in vascular tissue isolated from the rat, mouse, dog, pig, marmos et and cynomolgus monkey. *Br.J.Pharmacol*, Vol. 131, No. 7, (Dec 2000), pp.1262–1274, ISSN: 1476-5381

Doumas, M., Guo, D & Papademetriou, V. (2009).Carotid baroreceptor stimulation as a therapeutic target in hypertension and other cardiovascular conditions. *Expert Opin. Ther. Targets*, Vol.13, No.4, (Apr 2009), pp.413-425, ISSN: 1744-7631

Downham, MR. et al. (2003). Evaluation of two carrier protein angiotensin I conjugate vaccines to assess their future potential to control high blood pressure (hypertension) in man. *Br J Clin Pharmacol*, Vol.56, No.5, (Nov 2003), pp.505-12, ISSN: 1476-5381

Drummond, W. et al. (2007). Antihypertensive efficacy of the oral direct renin inhibitor aliskiren as add-on therapy in patients not responding to amlodipine monotherapy. *J Clin Hypertens*, Vol.9, No.10, (Oct 2007), pp.742-50, ISSN: 1751-7176

Ferrari, P. et al. (2006). Rostafuroxin: an ouabain antagonist that corrects renal and vascular Na+-K+-ATPase alterations in ouabain and adducin-dependent hypertension. *Am J Physiol Regul Integr Comp Physiol*, Vol.290, No. 3, (Mar 2006), pp.R529–R535, ISSN: 0363-6119

Fisher, JP. & Paton, JFR. (2011). The sympathetic nervous system and blood pressure in humans: implications for hypertension. *Journal of Human Hypertension*,(Jul 2011), pp.1–13, ISSN: 0950-9240

Gavazzi, G. et al. (2006). Decreased blood pressure in NOX1-deficient mice. *FEBS Lett*, Vol.580, No.2, (Jan 2006), pp.497–504, ISSN: 0014-5793

Goldblatt, H, Haas, E & Lamfrom, H. (1951). Antirenin in man and animals. *Trans Assoc Am Physicians*, Vol.64, (1951), pp.122-5, ISSN: 0066-9458

Guyton, AC, et al. (1972). Arterial pressure regulation: overriding dominance of the kidneys in long term regulation and in hypertension. *Am J Med*, Vol.52, No. 5, (May 1972), pp.584-94, ISSN: 0002-9343

Hamlyn, JM & Manunta, P. (2011).Endogenous Ouabain: A Link Between Sodium Intake and Hypertension. *Curr Hypertens Rep*, Vol.13, No. 1, (Feb 2011), pp.14–20, ISSN: 1534-3111

Hasenfuss, G. (2011). New Generation Barostim neo™ System. *Preliminary Results and Discussion, Proceedings of Symposium: Baroreflex Activation Therapy for Resistant Hypertension and Heart Failure at the European Society of Cardiology (ESC) Congress*, Paris, France, (Aug 2011)

Heusser, K. et al. (2010). Carotid baroreceptor stimulation, sympathetic activity, baroreflex function, and blood pressure in hypertensive patients. *Hypertension*, Vol.55, No.3, (Mar 2010), pp.619–626, ISSN: 1524-4563

Howlett, AC. (2002). The cannabinoid receptors. *Prostaglandins Other Lipid Media*, Vol. 68-69, (Aug 2002), pp. 619-31, ISSN: 1098-8823

Jahangir, A. & Terzic, A. (2005). K(ATP) channel therapeutics at the bedside. *J Mol Cell Cardiol.*, Vol. 39, No. 1, (Jul 2005), pp. 99-112, ISSN: 0022-2828

Jensen, LL, Harding, JW. Wright, JW. (1989). Increased blood pressure induced by central application of aminopeptidase inhibitors is angiotensinergic dependent in normotensive and hypertensive rat strains. *Brain Res Rev*, Vol. 490, No. 1, (Jun 1989), pp.48–55, ISSN: 0165-0173

Kearney, PM. et al. (2005). Global burden of hypertension: analysis of worldwide data. *Lancet*,Vol.365, No.9455,(Jan 2005), pp.217-23, ISSN: 0140-6736

Kowala, MC. et al. (2004). Novel Dual Action AT1 and ETA Receptor Antagonists Reduce Blood Pressure in Experimental Hypertension. *J Pharmacol Exp Ther*, Vol. 309, No.1, (Apr 2004), pp. 275-84, ISSN: 1521-0103

Krum, H. et al. (1998). The effect of an endothelin-receptor antagonist, Bosentan, on blood pressure in patients with essential hypertension. *N Engl J Med,* Vol. 338, No. 12, (Mar 1998), pp.784-90, ISSN: 0028-4793

Krum, H. et al. (2009). Catheter-based renal sympathetic denervation for resistant hypertension: a multicentre safety and proof-of-principle cohort study. *Lancet,* Vol. 373, No.9671, (Apr 2009), pp.1275-81, ISSN: 0140-6736

Lepicier, P. et al. (2006). Signaling pathways involved in the cardioprotective effects of cannabinoids. *J Pharmacol Sci,* Vol.102, No.2, (Oct 2006), pp.155-166, ISSN: 1347-8648

Lewis, EJ. et al. (2001). Renoprotective effect of the angiotensin-receptor antagonist irbesartan in patients with nephropathy due to type 2 diabetes. *N Engl J Med,* Vol. 345, No.12, (Sept 2001), pp.851–860, ISSN: 0028-4793

Liao, JK, Seto, M & Noma, K. (2007). Rho Kinase (ROCK) Inhibitors. *J Cardiovasc Pharmacol,* Vol.50, No.1, (Jul 2007), pp.17–24, ISSN: 1533-4023

Liu, Q. et al. (1999). Identification of urotensin II as the endogenous ligand for the orphan G protein coupled receptor GPR14. *Biochem. Biophys. Res. Commun,* Vol. 266, No.1, (Dec 1999), pp. 174–178, ISSN: 0006-291X

Maguire, JJ. et al. (2004). Cellular distribution of immuno reactive urotensin II in human tissues with evidence of increased expression in atherosclerosis and a greater constrictor response of small compared to large coronary arteries. *Peptides,* Vol. 25, No. 10, (Oct 2004), pp.1767–1774, ISSN: 0196-9781

Manunta, P. et al. (2009). Endogenous ouabain in cardiovascular function and disease. *J Hypertens,* Vol. 27, No.1, (Jan 2009), pp.9-18, ISSN: 1473-5598

Masumoto, A. et al. (2001). Possible involvement of Rho-kinase in the patogénesis of hypertension in humans. *Hypertension,* Vol. 38, No. 6, (Dec 2001), pp.1307–1310, ISSN: 1524-4563

Matsuno, K. et al. (2005). Nox1 is involved in angiotensin II-mediated hypertension: a study in Nox1-deficient mice. *Circulation,* Vol.112, No. 17, (Oct 2005), pp.2677–2685, ISSN: 1524-4539

Matsushita, M. et al. (2001).Co expression of urotensin II and its receptor (GPR14) in human cardiovascular and renal tissues. *J. Hypertens,* Vol.19, No.12, (Dec 2001), pp.2185–2190, ISSN: 1473-5598

McMurray, J. et al. for the Aliskiren Observation of Heart Failure Treatment (ALOFT) Investigators. (2008). Effects of the oral direct renin inhibitor aliskiren in patients with symptomatic heart failure. *Circ Heart Fail,* Vol.1, No.1, (May 2008), pp.17-24, ISSN: 1941-3297

Michel, JB. et al. (1987). Active immunization against renin in normotensive marmoset. *Proc Natl Acad Sci USA,* Vol.84, No.12, (Jun 1987), pp.4346-50, ISSN: 1091-6490

Mitrovic, V. et al. (1991). Hemodynamic and neurohumoral effects of moxonidine in patients with essential hypertension. *Cardiovasc Drugs Ther,* Vol.5, No.6, (Dec 1991), pp.967-972, ISSN: 1755-5922

Morales Olivas, FJ. & Estañ Yago, L. (2010). Conceptos nuevos sobre el sistema renina angiotensina. *Hipertens riesgo vasc,* Vol.27, No.5, (May 2010), pp.211–217, ISSN: 1889-1837

Moreau, C. et al.(2000). The molecular basis of the specificity of action of K(ATP) channel openers. *EMBO J,* Vol. 19, No.24, (Dec 2000), pp. 6644-51, ISSN: 0261-4189

Morrissey, DM, Brookes, VS & Cooke, WT. (1953). Sympathectomy in the treatment of hypertension; review of 122 cases. *Lancet,* Vol.1, No.6757, (Feb 1953), pp.403–408, ISSN: 0140-6736

Nickenig, G. (2004). Should Angiotensin II Receptor Blockers and Statins Be Combined? *Circulation,* Vol.110, No.8, (Aug 2004), pp.1013-1020, ISSN: 1524-4539

Nussberger, J. et al. (2002). Angiotensin II suppression in humans by the orally active renin inhibitor Aliskiren (SPP100): comparison with enalapril. *Hypertension,* Vol.39, No.1, (Jan 2002), pp.E1-8, ISSN: 1524-4563

Ondetti, MA, Rubin, B & Cushman, DW. (1977). MA, Design of specific inhibitors of angiotensin-converting enzyme: new class of orally active antihypertensive agents. *Science,* Vol. 196, No.4288, (Apr 1977), pp.441-4, ISSN: 0036-8075

Pacher, P. et al. (2008). Modulation of the Endocannabinoid System in Cardiovascular Disease Therapeutic Potential and Limitations. *Hypertension,* Vol. 52, No. 4, (Oct 2008), pp. 601-7, ISSN: 0194-911X

Parsonnet, V. et al. (1969). Electrical stimulation of the carotid sinus nerve. *Surg Clin North Am,* Vol.49, No.3, (Jun 1969), pp.589-596, ISSN: 0039-6109

Parving, HH. et al, for the AVOID Study Investigators.(2008). Aliskiren combined with losartan in type 2 diabetes and nephropathy. *N Engl J Med,* Vol.358, No. 23, (Jun 2008), pp.2433-46, ISSN: 0028-4793

Pfeffer, MA. et al. (2003). Valsartan, captopril, or both in myocardial infarction complicated by heart failure, left ventricular dysfunction, or both. *N Engl J Med,* Vol. 349, No.20, (Nov 2003), pp.1893–1906, ISSN: 0028-4793

Pillion, G et al. (1994). Long-term control of blood pressure by rilmenidine in high-risk populations. *Am J Cardiol,* Vol. 74, No.13, (Dec 1994), pp.58A-65A, ISSN: 0002-9149

Rikitake, Y. & Liao, JK. (2005). ROCKs as therapeutic targets in cardiovascular diseases. *Expert Rev Cardiovasc Ther,* Vol. 3, No. 3, (May 2005), pp. 441–451, ISSN: 1477-9072

Rothfeld, EL. et al. (1969). The effect of carotid sinus nerve stimulation on cardiovascular dynamics in man. *Angiology,* Vol.20, No.4,(Apr 1969),pp.213-218,ISSN: 0003-3197

Ruilope, LM. et al. (2010). Blood-pressure reduction with LCZ696, a novel dual-acting inhibitor of the angiotensin II receptor and neprilysin: a randomised, double-blind, placebo-controlled, active comparator study. *Lancet,* Vol. 375, No.9722, (Apr 2010), pp.1255–66, ISSN: 0140-6736

Sagnella, GA. (2002).Vasopeptidase inhibitors. *Journal of Renin Angiotensin Aldosterone System,* Vol. 3, No. 2, (Jun 2002), pp.90-95, ISSN: 1752-8976

Sandhiya, S. & Dkhar, SA. (2009). Potassium channels in health, disease & development of channel modulators. *Indian J Med Res,* Vol. 129, No. 3, (Mar 2009), pp. 223-32, ISSN: 0019-5359

Scheffers, I., Kroon, AA. & de Leeuw, P. (2008). Renal hemodynamics during chronic therapy with electrical stimulation of the carotid sinus in humans. *J Hypertens,* Vol.26, Suppl 1, (2008), pp.S465, ISSN: 0952-1178

Scheffers, I. et al. (2008). Sustained blood pressure reduction by baroreflex hypertension therapy with a chronically implanted system: 2-years data from the Rheos DEBUT-HT study in patients with resistant hypertension. *J Hypertens,* Vol.26, Suppl 1, (2008), pp.S19, ISSN: 0952-1178

Schoner, W. (2002). Endogenous cardiac glycosides, a new class of steroid hormones. *Eur. J. Biochem,* Vol. 269,No. 10, (May 2002), pp. 2440–8, ISSN: 1742-4658

Schoner, W & Scheiner Bobis G. (2008). Role of endogenous cardiotonic steroids in sodium homeostasis. *Nephrol Dial Transplant*, Vol.23, No. 9, (Sept 2008), pp.2723–2729, ISSN: 1460-2385

Selden, R, Smith, TW & Findley, W.(1972). Ouabain Pharmacokinetics in Dog and Man: Determination by Radioimmunoassay. *Circulation*, Vol. 45, No. 6, (Jun 1972), pp. 1176-82, ISSN: 1524-4539

Shepherd, J. et al. (1995). Prevention of coronary heart disease with pravastatin in men with hypercholesterolemia: West of Scotland coronary prevention study group. *N Engl J Med*, Vol. 333, No.20, (Nov 1995), pp.1301–1307, ISSN: 0028-4793

Sica, D.et al. (2006). Aliskiren, a novel renin inhibitor, is well tolerated and has sustained BP lowering effects alone or in combination with HCTZ during long term (52 weeks) treatment of hypertension. *Eur Heart J*, Vol.27 Suppl 1 (Sept 2006), Abstract P797, ISSN: 1522-9645

Solomon, SD. et al. (2009). Effect of the direct Renin inhibitor aliskiren, the Angiotensin receptor blocker losartan, or both on left ventricular mass in patients with hypertension and left ventricular hypertrophy. *Circulation*, Vol.119, No.4, (Feb 2009), pp.530-7, ISSN: 1524-4539

Staessen, JA. et al.(2011). Main results of the Ouabain and Adducin for Specific Intervention on Sodium in Hypertension Trial (OASIS-HT): a randomized placebo controlled phase 2 dose finding study of rostafuroxin. *Trials*, Vol.12, No.13, (Jan 2011), pp.1-14, ISSN: 1745-6215

Stocker, R & Keaney, JF, Jr (2004). Role of oxidative modifications in atherosclerosis. *Physiol Rev*, Vol.84, No.4, (Oct 2004), pp.1381–1478, ISSN: 1522-1210

Suguro, T. et al. (2007). Increased human urotensin II levels are correlated with carotid atherosclerosis in essential hypertension. *Am.J. Hypertens*, Vol.20, No.2, (Feb 2007), pp.211–217, ISSN: 0895-7061

Susic, D. et al. (2004). Cardiovascular and renal effects of a collagen cross link breaker (ALT 711) in adult and aged spontaneously hypertensive rats. *Am J Hypertens*, Vol.17, No.4, (Apr 2004), pp.328–333, ISSN: 0895-7061

Timmermans, PB, et al. (1991).The discovery of a new class of highly specific nonpeptide angiotensin II receptor antagonists. *Am J Hypertens*, Vol. 4, No.4 Pt 2, (Apr 1991), pp.275S-281S, ISSN: 0895-7061

Tissot, AC. et al. (2008). Effect of immunisation with CYT006-AngQb against angiotensin II on ambulatory blood pressure: a double-blind randomised placebo controlled phase IIa study. *Lancet*, Vol.371, No.9615, (Mar 2008), pp.821–27, ISSN: 0140-6736

Trapani, AJ. et al. (2004). CGS 35601 and its Orally Active Prodrug CGS 37808 as Triple Inhibitors of Endothelin-converting Enzyme-1, Neutral Endopeptidase 24.11, and Angiotensin converting Enzyme. *J Cardiovasc Pharmacol*, Vol.44, Suppl 1, (Nov 2004), pp.S211-5, ISSN: 1533-4023

Tsoukas, P, Kane, E & Giaid, A. (2011). Potential clinical implications of the urotensin II receptor antagonists. *Frontiers in Pharmacology*, Vol.2, No.38, (Jul 2011), pp.1-11, ISSN: 1663-9812

Tuckman, J. et al. (1972). Evaluation of carotid sinus nerve stimulation in the treatment of hypertension. *Ther Umsch*, Vol.29, No.6, (Jun 1972), pp.382–391, ISSN: 0040-5930

Van Zwieten, PA. (1996). Modulation of sympathetic outflow by centrally actino antihypertensive drugs. *Cardiovasc Drugs Ther*, Vol. 10, suppl 1, (Jun 1996), pp.283-289, ISSN: 1755-5922

Vlassara, H. & Palace, MR. (2002). Diabetes and advanced glycation endproducts. *J Intern Med*, Vol.251, No.2, (Feb 2002), pp.87–101, ISSN: 1365-2796

Voskuil, M. et al. (2011). Percutaneous renal denervation for the treatment of resistant essential hypertension; the first Dutch experience. *Neth Heart J*, Vol. 19. No. 7-8, (Aug 2011), pp. 319–23, ISSN: 1876-6250

Wang, H, Long, CL. & Zhang, YL. (2004). A new ATP sensitive potassium channel opener reduces blood pressure and reverses cardiovascular remodeling in experimental hypertension.*The Journal of Pharmacology and Experimental Therapeutics*,Vol. 312, No. 3,(Nov 2004),pp.1326-1333, ISSN: 1521-0103

Wang, H, Long, CL. & Zhang, YL. (2005). A new ATP-sensitive potassium channel opener reduces blood pressure and reverses cardiovascular remodeling in experimental hypertension. *J Pharmacol Exp Ther*, Vol. 312, No. 3, (Mar 2005), pp.1326-33, ISSN: 0022-3565

Wang, H. et al. (2007). A new ATP sensitive potassium channel opener protects endothelial function in cultured aortic endothelial cells. *Cardiovasc Res*, Vol.73, No.3, (Feb 2007), pp.497–503, ISSN: 1755-3245

Weir, MR. et al. (2007). Antihypertensive efficacy, safety and tolerability of the oral direct renin inhibitor aliskiren in patients with hypertension: a pooled analysis. *J Am Soc Hypertens*, Vol.1, No.4, (Jul-Aug 2007), pp.264-77, ISSN: 1933-1711

Wheal, AJ. et al. (2007). Cardiovascular effects of cannabinoids in conscious spontaneously hypertensive rats. *Br J Pharmacol*, Vol.152, No.5, (Nov 2007), pp.717-724, ISSN: 1476-5381

Wind, S. et al. (2010). Comparative pharmacology of chemically distinct NADPH oxidase inhibitors. *British Journal of Pharmacology*, Vol.161, No. 4, (Oct 2010), pp.885–898, ISSN: 1476-5381

Witkowski, A. et al.(2011). Effects of Renal Sympathetic Denervation on Blood Pressure, Sleep Apnea Course, and Glycemic Control in Patients With Resistant Hypertension and Sleep Apnea. *Hypertension*,Vol. 58, No. 4, (Oct 2011), pp. 559-65, ISSN: 1524-4563

Wood, JM. et al. (2003). Structure-based design of aliskiren, a novel orally effective renin inhibitor. *Biochem Biophys Res Commun*, Vol.308, No.4, (Sept 2003), pp.698-705, ISSN: 0006-291X

Wright, J.W., Harding, J.W., 1992. Regulatory role of brain angiotensins in the control of physiological and behavioral responses. *Brain Res. Rev*, Vol.17, No.3, (Sep-Dec 1992), pp.227–262, ISSN: 0165-0173

Wright, J.W., Harding, J.W. (1994). Brain angiotensin receptor subtypes in the control of physiological and behavioral responses. *Neurosci. Biobehav. Rev*, Vol.18, No.1, (Spring 1994), pp.21–53, ISSN: 0149-7634

Wright, J.W., Harding, J.W. (1997). Important roles for angiotensin III and IV in the brain renin angiotensin system. *Brain Res. Rev*, Vol. 25, No.1, (Sept 1997), pp.96–124, ISSN: 0165-0173

Yu, A & Frishman, WH. (1996). Imidazoline receptor agonist drugs: a new approach to the treatment of systemic hypertension. *J Clin Pharmacol*, Vol. 36, No.2, (Feb 1997), pp. 98-111, ISSN: 1552-4604

Zhu, Y.C., Zhu, Y.Z., & Moore, P.K. (2006). The role of urotensin II in cardiovascular and renal physiology and diseases. *Br.J.Pharmacol*, Vol.148, No.7, (Aug 2006).pp. 884-901, ISSN: 1476-5381

2

Dual L/N-Type Ca^{2+} Channel Blocker: Cilnidipine as a New Type of Antihypertensive Drug

Akira Takahara
Toho University,
Japan

1. Introduction

Cilnidipine is a unique dihydropyridine derivative Ca^{2+} channel blocker with an inhibitory action on the sympathetic N-type Ca^{2+} channels (Uneyama et al., 1999a). It has been clarified that cilnidipine exerts antisympathetic actions in various examinations from cell to human levels. Furthermore, its renoprotective, neuroprotective and cardioprotective effects have been demonstrated in clinical practice or animal examinations. After the introduction of nifedipine, many Ca^{2+} channel blockers with long-lasting action have been synthesized to decline sympathetic reflex during antihypertensive therapy. Based on each pharmacokinetic profile, Ca^{2+} channel blockers have been divided into three groups; namely, 1st, 2nd, and 3rd generation. Since cilnidipine directly inhibits the sympathetic neurotransmitter release by N-type Ca^{2+} channel-blocking property, the drug can be expected as 4th generation, providing an effective strategy for the treatment of cardiovascular diseases (Takahara, 2009).

Recently, cilnidipine has been demonstrated to suppress renin-angiotensin-aldosterone system at anti-hypertensive doses in animal examinations, whereas other Ca^{2+} channel blockers usually activates such vasopressor system after acute or repeated administrations. Interestingly, antihypertensive therapies with angiotensin II receptor blockers sometimes activate renin-angiotensin system, which is effectively suppressed by cilnidipine. This may provide synergistic and effective therapeutic strategies during combined administration of cilnidipine and angiotensin II receptor blockers. The possible mechanisms to suppress renin-angiotensin-aldosterone system appear to be clarified. In human adrenocortical cells, where N-type Ca^{2+} channels are recently found to act as a source of intracellular Ca^{2+} mobilization, cilnidipine as well as a specific N-type Ca^{2+} channel blocker ω-conotoxin effectively inhibits angiotensin II-induced aldosterone synthesis.

In this chapter, we introduce a pharmacological profile of cilnidipine in combined with its clinical antihypertensive and anti-sympathetic actions. We further review utilities of cilnidipine for management of hypertension and its complications through inhibition of sympathetic N-type Ca^{2+} channels and renin-angiotensin-aldosterone system.

2. Ca^{2+} channels: Physiological role and pharmacological modification

Rise in intracellular Ca^{2+} triggers a variety of physiological processes, and there are many channels and pumps involved in controlling intracellular Ca^{2+} level. Among them, voltage-gated Ca^{2+} channels play a key role in this process, which is a pharmacological target molecule for so-called Ca^{2+} channel blockers. In excitatory cells such as smooth and cardiac muscle cells and neurons, high voltage-activated (HVA) Ca^{2+} channels are well known to regulate a variety of cellular events, which include muscle contraction, neuronal electrical activity, the release of neurotransmitters and hormones as well as gene expressions. On the other hand, low voltage-activated (LVA) Ca^{2+} channels are expressed throughout the body, including nervous tissue, heart, kidney, smooth muscle and many endocrine organs. The channels in the brain are considered to be involved in repetitive low threshold firing and nociception. In the heart, they are expressed in the sino-atrial node and are considered to participate in cardiac pacemaking (Tanaka & Shigenobu, 2005).

2.1 Classification of Ca^{2+} channels

Ca^{2+} channels are classified into at least 6 subtypes; namely, L-, N-, P-, Q-, R-, and T-type, based on electrophysiological and pharmacological evidences (Varadi et al., 1995). The T-type Ca^{2+} channels are known as low-voltage-activated Ca^{2+} channels that activate and deactivate slowly, but inactivate rapidly. The other five types of Ca^{2+} channels are all high-voltage-activated Ca^{2+} channels, which depolarize at approximately –40 mV. Molecular biological techniques have shown that Ca^{2+} channels are composed of α_1, α_2-δ, β, and γ subunits using L-type Ca^{2+} channels from skeletal muscles. In particular, the α_1 subunit forms the Ca^{2+} transmission pore, which fulfills the most important function. Furthermore, 10 α_1 subunits have been cloned and classified into 3 subfamilies: Cav1.x; Cav2.x; and Cav3.x, based on their gene sequence similarity (Catterall et al., 2003). More importantly, the α_1 subunit has a binding site for Ca^{2+} channel blockers.

2.2 Ca^{2+} channels in the cardiovascular system

In the cardiovascular system, L-type Ca^{2+} channels are predominantly expressed in the heart and vessels, which regulate cardiac contractility, sinus nodal function and vascular tone. β-adrenergic stimulation enhances the force of cardiac contraction through activation of cAMP-mediated activation of protein kinase A that in turn increases the L-type Ca^{2+} channel currents, causing a greater rate of release of Ca^{2+} from the sarcoplasmic reticulum. In the arterial vessels, receptor stimulation or membrane depolarization activates Ca^{2+} influx through Ca^{2+} channels and myosin light chain kinase, leading to smooth muscle contraction. Thus, L-type Ca^{2+} channels have been recognized as a pharmacological target for the treatment of cardiovascular disease. Most of Ca^{2+} channel blockers are well known to have selectivity for vascular tissues rather than cardiac function. On the other hand, verapamil, diltiazem and bepridil have been shown to possess less vascular selectivity, which are used for supraventricular and/or ventricular arrhythmias. The selectivity of Ca^{2+} channel blockers for cardiac and vascular actions may be associated with that the membrane potential in vascular smooth muscle cells is definitely less negative than the diastolic membrane potential of working cardiac muscle cells. In the vascular system, arterioles appear to be more sensitive to Ca^{2+} channel blockers than venules; orthostatic hypotension is not a common adverse effect.

2.3 Ca^{2+} channels in the sympathetic nerve system

The most thoroughly characterized role of Ca^{2+} in the nerve is the triggering of exocytosis. The synaptic vesicle cycles at nerve endings could be divided into the following processes:

a) translocation of the synaptic vesicle filled with norepinephrine and epinephrine to the active zone; b) docking at the active zone and priming; c) fusion triggered by Ca^{2+} and exocytosis; d) endocytosis of empty synaptic vesicle to become coated vesicles; e) endosome fusion and budding to make the synaptic vesicle re-generation; and f) the neurotransmitters uptake to the regenerated synaptic vesicle. Entered Ca^{2+} through voltage-gated Ca^{2+} channels bind to synaplotagmin, changing the conformation of a large protein superfamily called as SNARE complexes (formed by 4 α-helices; synaptobrevin, synaptotagmin, syntaxin and SNAP 25), leading to fusion of vesicle membrane into plasma membrane. At these steps, the N-type Ca^{2+} channel plays an important role as a Ca^{2+} supplier. More than 60 Ca^{2+} channels open for each vesicle for rapid release (Uneyama et al., 1999).

In the sympathetic nervous systems, N-type Ca^{2+} channels are localized at the nerve endings. Using a patch clamp method, N-type Ca^{2+} channels are shown to contribute about 85% of all other types of Ca^{2+} channels in the sympathetic neuronal cells. N-type Ca^{2+} channels have been demonstrated to predominantly regulate norepinephrine release in the superior cervical ganglia neurons using a selective N-type Ca^{2+} channel blocker ω-conotoxin GVIA (Hirning et al., 1988). This finding was further supported by subsequent experiments using isolated rat arterial preparations. In a clinical study, systemic administration of ω-conotoxin MVIIA (SNX-111) has been shown to induce sympatholytic action.

2.4 Ca^{2+} channels in the adrenal gland

Chromaffin cells in the medulla of the adrenal gland are innervated by the splanchnic nerve and secrete catecholamines into the blood stream. In anesthetized dogs, the splanchnic nerve stimulation increased the catecholamine secretion from adrenal gland, which was effectively inhibited by an N-type Ca^{2+} channel blocker ω-conotoxin GVIA but not by L-type Ca^{2+} channel blockers nifedipine or verapamil (Kimura et al., 1994). Many in vitro studies also support that N-type Ca^{2+} channels are localized at chromaffin cells to regulate the release of catecholamine. Recently, it is shown that N-type Ca^{2+} channels are also localized at the human adrenocortical cells, playing an important role in the secretion of adrenocortical hormones (Aritomi et al., 2011a). Furthermore, N-type Ca^{2+} channels may offer the different way of controlling corticosteroid production in adrenocortical cells than other types of voltage-gated Ca^{2+} channels.

3. New generation Ca^{2+} channel blocker: Cilnidipine

Cilnidipine is a unique dihydropyridine derivative L-type Ca^{2+} channel blocker with an inhibitory action on the sympathetic N-type Ca^{2+} channels. As shown in Fig. 1, Ca^{2+} channels are ordinarily activated by membrane depolarization in the vascular cells or sympathetic neurons, leading to vascular contraction or neurotransmitter releases. During antihypertensive therapies with pure L-type Ca^{2+} channel blockers like nifedipine, the sympathetic reflex is sometimes occurred due to hypotension, leading to activation of sympathetic N-type Ca^{2+} channels, which induces several cardiovascular responses including vascular contraction, tachycardia and renin secretion (Takahara 2009). Cilnidipine can directly inhibit the sympathetic neurotransmitter release by its N-type Ca^{2+} channel-blocking property, which may reduce risk of cardiovascular diseases closely associated with sympathetic nerve activation. The wide variety of pharmacological actions of cilnidipine has been investigated, which is summarized in Table 1.

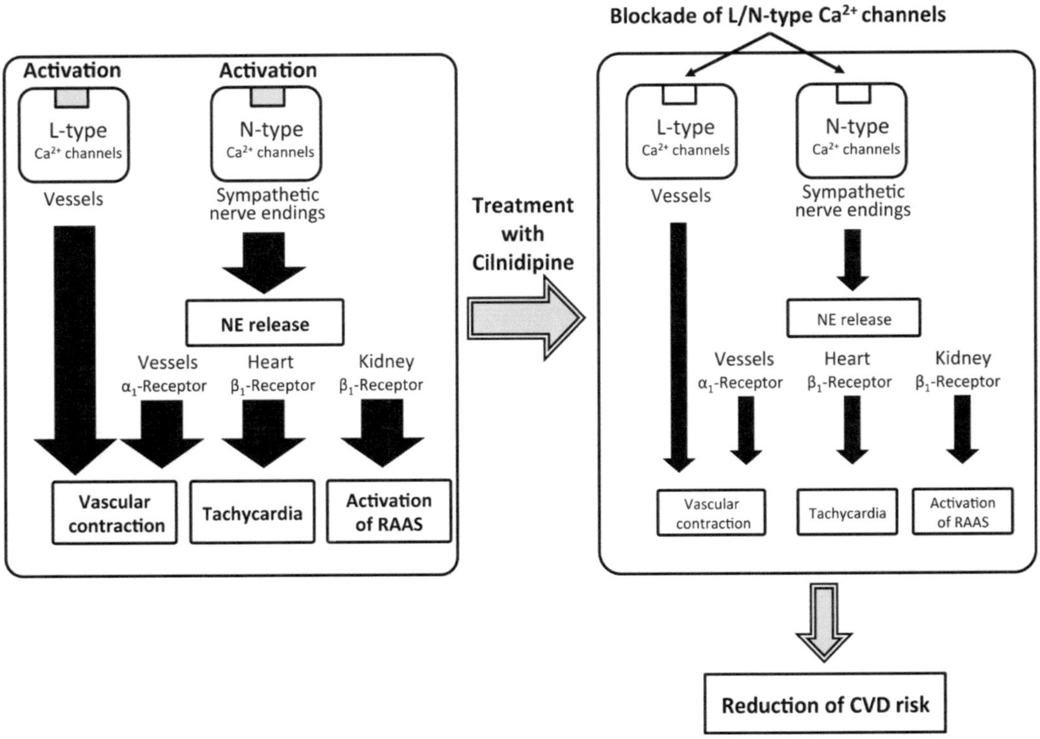

Fig. 1. Diagrammatic representation of L/N-type dual action of cilnidipine. Cilnidipine directly inhibits the sympathetic neurotransmitter (norepinephrine; NE) release by N-type Ca^{2+} channel-blocking property in addition to vascular L-type Ca^{2+} channel inhibition, leading to suppression of renin-angiotensin-aldosterone system (RAAS). Thus, the drug can be expected to provide an effective strategy for the treatment of cardiovascular diseases (CVD).

3.1 Pharmacology

L-type Ca^{2+} channel-blocking actions of cilnidipine were widely examined in earlier experimental studies, showing that its potency was greater than that of nifedipine. In 1997, N-type Ca^{2+} channel-blocking action was found in cilnidipine (Uneyama et al., 1997). Submicromolecular concentrations of cilnidipine effectively suppressed N-type Ca^{2+} channel currents in isolated sympathetic neurons. The inhibitory effect of various dihydropyridines on cardiac L-type Ca^{2+} channels was further compared in isolated ventricular myocytes with that on N-type Ca^{2+} channels in superior cervical ganglion neurons of the rat (Uneyama et al., 1999b). In that study, all dihydropyridines, except cilnidipine, showed a small inhibitory effect at a concentration of 1 μM. The N-type channel-blocking action of cilnidipine has also been confirmed in IMR-32 human neuroblastoma cells and PC12 pheochromocytoma of the rat adrenal medulla cells. Furthermore, it has been demonstrated that the N-type Ca^{2+} channel-blocking effects of cilnidipine leading to anti-sympathetic action can be observed at its anti-hypertensive doses (Takahara et al., 2002).

Mode of action	Inhibition of L-type Ca^{2+} channels (vascular smooth muscle, in vitro); inhibition of N-type Ca^{2+} channels (sympathetic neuron, in vitro)
Pharmacology	
1) Cardiovascular action	Vascular relaxation (in vitro); hypotensive action (in vivo)
2) Anti-sympathetic action	Decrease of catecholamine release, tissue (kidney) norepinephrine level, (in vitro, in vivo); inhibition of sympathetic tachycardia and cold stress-induced vasoconstriction (in vivo); decrease in plasma/urinary norepinephrine, muscle sympathetic nerve activity, low frequency/high frequency ratio (LF/HF ratio), and plasma level of ß-thromboglobulin (clinical)
3) Suppression of renin-angiotensin-aldosterone system	Decrease in plasma level of angiotensin II and aldosterone (in vivo, clinical); inhibition of aldosterone production (adrenocortical cells, in vitro); inhibition of reflex aldosterone production, and angiotensin II-renin feedback (in vivo)
4) Anti-oxidation	Inhibition of NADPH oxidase-derived superoxide production (kidney, in vivo)
5) Others	Improvement of insulin resistance (in vivo); increases of nitric oxide production (in vitro); protection from retinal neuronal injury (in vivo); anti-nociception (in vivo)
Antihypertensive action	
1) Animal model	Antihypertensive action in spontaneously hypertensive rats, stroke-prone spontaneously hypertensive rat, renal hypertensive rats, DOCA-salt hypertensive rats, Otsuka Long-Evans Tokushima Fatty rat, Dahl salt sensitive rat and 2-kidney 1-clip hypertensive dogs (in vivo)
2) Human	Essential hypertension; severe hypertension; hypertension with chronic kidney disease, cerebrovascular disease or diabetes (clinical)
Actions in key organs	
1) Kidney	Increase in renal blood flow; dilation of afferent and efferent arterioles; natriuresis; inhibition of renal nerve stimulation-induced antinatriuresis; suppression of albuminuria; glomerular hypertrophy and interstitial fibrosis; decrease in renal angiotensin II content (in vivo); decrease in albuminuria and urinary protein (clinical)
2) Heart	Increase in coronary blood flow (in vitro, in vivo); suppression of vasopressin-induced ST depression; reduction of the myocardial infarct size and incidence of ventricular premature beats after ischemia-reperfusion; abbreviation of abnormally prolonged ventricular repolarization (in vivo); decrease in BNP, LV mass index, heart rate and cardiothoracic ratio (clinical)
3) Brain	Downward shift of the lower limit of autoregulation for cerebral blood flow; reduction of the cerebral infarction size (in vivo); increase in cerebral blood flow (clinical)

Table 1. Summary of pharmacological effects of cilnidipine

3.2 Antihypertensive action

In animal examinations, cilnidipine has a slow-onset and long-lasting antihypertensive action in spontaneously hypertensive rats, renal hypertensive rats, DOCA-salt hypertensive rats, and 2-kidney 1-clip hypertensive dogs. In addition, cilnidipine significantly decreases the blood pressure of stroke-prone spontaneously hypertensive rats (Watanabe et al. 1995a) and Dahl salt-sensitive rats (Aritomi et al., 2010).

In clinical studies, the antihypertensive effect of cilnidipine has been demonstrated in hypertensive patients, and also in patients with severe hypertension or with complications such as chronic kidney disease, cerebrovascular disease and diabetes. Cilnidipine has been reported to improve some hypertensive conditions closely associated with sympathetic nerve activation such as morning hypertension, nocturnal hypertension, white-coat phenomenon, mental stress and cold stress (Yamagishi, 2006).

3.3 Anti-sympathetic action

The anti-sympathetic action of cilnidipine has been demonstrated in several experimental studies; increases in the heart rate and plasma catecholamine level induced by cold stress, hypotension or spinal nerve stimulation of the rat were effectively suppressed by cilnidipine but not other Ca^{2+} channel blockers (Uneyama et al., 1999a). Importantly, the N-type Ca^{2+} channel-blockade hardly affects parasympathetic neurotransmission (Konda et al., 2001). We compared effects of 4 Ca^{2+} channel blockers (nifedipine, amlodipine, azelnidipine and cilnidipine) on hypotension-induced sympathetic activation in the halothane-anesthetized canine model (Fig. 2, Takahara et al., 2007; Ishizaka et al., 2010). Intravenous infusion of nifedipine or amlodipine decreased the mean blood pressure with increments of heart rate and cardiac contractility. Azelnidipine also deceased the mean blood pressure with an increment of cardiac contractility whereas marked tachycardia was not induced, which is in accordance with a previous report showing its direct suppressive effects on sinus nodal automaticity. On the other hand, no significant change in the heart rate or cardiac contractility was observed after intravenous infusion of cilnidipine. These results strongly indicate that cilnidipine is desirable among Ca^{2+} channel blockers to minimize reflex sympathetic nerve activation.

Similar actions of cilnidipine can be observed in the clinical investigations using a parameter of plasma/urinary norepinephrine, ^{123}I-metaiodobenzylguanidine (MIBG), muscle sympathetic nerve activity, low frequency/high frequency ratio (LF/HF ratio) or heart rate, each of which help us better understand their clinical effects on sympathetic nerve activity (Takahara 2009). More importantly, a clinical study of cold pressor test has shown that cilnidipine decreased plasma level of ß-thromboglobulin, a marker of platelet activation, which may prevent arterial thrombosis formation associated with increased sympathetic tone.

3.4 Renal action

There are observations that L-type Ca^{2+} channel blockers, such as verapamil, nicardipine, felodipine and nifedipine, induce renal vasodilation and natriuresis in anesthetized dogs and rats. Similarly, cilnidipine increases the renal blood flow and urinary Na^{+} excretion without affecting creatinine clearance in dogs (Takahara et al., 1997). The kidney is densely innervated by adrenergic nerve fibers. The renal nerve stimulation releases norepinephrine and induces renal vasoconstriction, anti-natriuresis and renin secretion via activation of adrenoceptors in the vascular vessels, renal tubular cells and granular cells of the juxtaglomerular apparatus, respectively, which cannot be suppressed by typical L-type Ca^{2+} channel blockers in several experimental studies (Ogasawara et al., 1993). On the other hand, it has been demonstrated that these responses to renal nerve stimulation are suppressed by natriuretic doses of cilnidipine via its N-type Ca^{2+} channel blocking property.

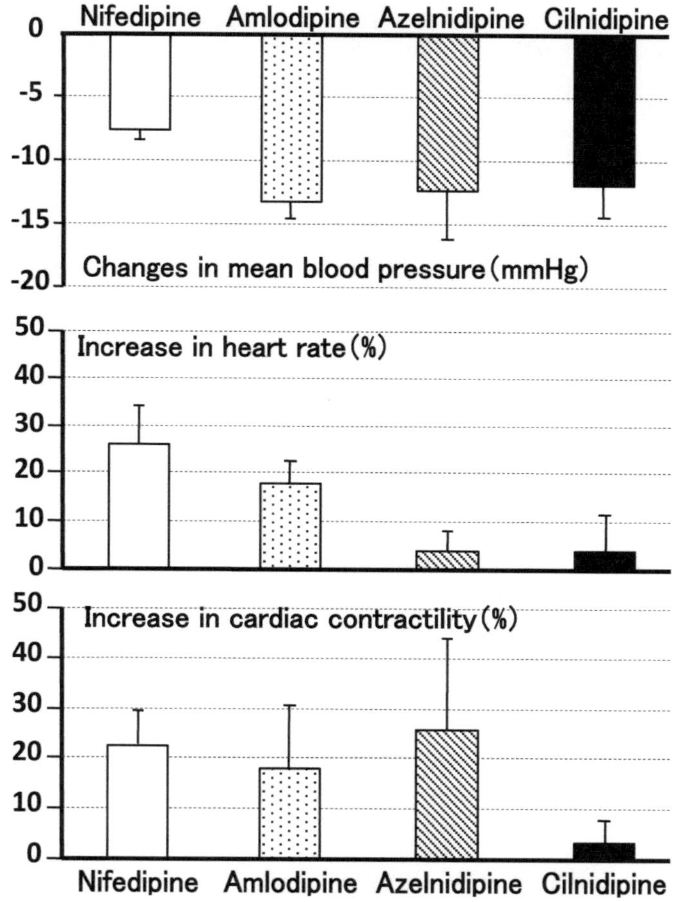

Fig. 2. Comparison of effects of Ca^{2+} channel blockers on hypotension-induced sympathetic activation. Nifedipine, amlodipine, azelnidipine or cilnidipine was intravenously administered to halothane-anesthetized dogs, and changes in mean blood pressure, heart rate and cardiac contractility were observed. The intravenous doses of nifedipine, amlodipine, azelnidipine and cilnidipine used were 3, 200, 70 and 3 μg/kg, respectively. Values are expressed as means±SE. Data are quoted and modified from Takahara et al., 2007 and Ishizaka et al., 2010.

Glomerular filtration is essentially regulated by afferent and efferent arterial tone. Since sensitivity of Ca^{2+} channel blockers to afferent and efferent arteries varies, Ca^{2+} channel blockers should be appropriately selected for hypertensive patients with chronic kidney disease. Since the sympathetic nerves are distributed to the afferent and efferent arteries, N-type Ca^{2+} channel-blocking activity may be partly associated with control of the glomerular pressure. Indeed, cilnidipine has been demonstrated to dilate both afferent and efferent arteries using the hydronephrotic kidney model of the rat (Konno & Kimura, 2008). Furthermore, in renal injury animal models, cilnidipine reduces glomerular capillary pressure, afferent and efferent arteriolar resistances, urinary albumin excretion, and glomerular volume as well as plasma norepinephrine levels.

In clinical studies, cilnidipine significantly decreased urinary albumin excretion without affecting serum creatinine concentration in hypertensive patients, which is comparable to the angiotensin-converting enzyme inhibitor benazepril. Other studies have shown that the renal protective effect of cilnidipine was greater than that of pure L-type Ca^{2+} channel blockers. Furthermore, the combination of cilnidipine and valsartan was shown to decrease the albumin/creatinine ratio more markedly than valsartan alone. Recently, the multi-center, open-labeled and randomized trial of Cilnidipine versus Amlodipine Randomized Trial for Evaluation in Renal disease (CARTER) has shown that cilnidipine is superior to amlodipine in preventing the progression of proteinuria in patients with hypertension and chronic renal disease when coupled with a renin–angiotensin system inhibitor (Fujita et al., 2007).

3.5 Cardiovascular action

Since the first generation of Ca^{2+} channel blockers were known to suppress cardiac functions such as contractility, sino-atrial automaticity, and atrioventricular conduction at vasodilator doses, pharmaceutical companies have developed new Ca^{2+} channel blockers with higher vascular selectivity in addition to slow kinetics as a new generation. The blood-perfused canine heart preparation is an excellent model to quantitatively determine cardio-vascular selectivity of Ca^{2+} channel blockers, and many Ca^{2+} channel blockers were analyzed using this model (Taira, 1987). Cilnidipine has about 10 times more potent coronary vasodilator action and higher vascular selectivity than nifedipine in this heart preparation. An in vivo experimental study has confirmed that cilnidipine shows anti-anginal effects in the vasopressin-induced angina model (Saitoh et al., 2003). A recent study indicates that cilnidipine relaxes human arteries through Ca^{2+} channel antagonism and increases production of nitric oxide by enhancement of endothelial nitric oxide synthase in the human internal thoracic artery (Fan et al., 2011).

The cardioprotective action of cilnidipine against ischemia has been analyzed in a rabbit model of myocardial infarction, in which cilnidipine decreased the myocardial interstitial norepinephrine levels during ischemia and reperfusion periods, leading to reduction of the myocardial infarct size and incidence of ventricular premature beats (Nagai et al., 2005). Clinically, cilnidipine has been reported to improve left ventricular diastolic function in patients with hypertensive heart disease (Kosaka et al., 2009). These cardioprotective actions are probably associated with suppression of cardiac sympathetic overactivity via blockade of N-type Ca^{2+} channels and/or anti-oxidative (as described below) effects of cilnidipine, which should be further clarified.

3.6 Cerebrovascular action

The brain is known to have an autoregulatory capacity that allows cerebral blood vessels to maintain constant cerebral blood flow by dilating or contracting in response to abrupt changes in blood pressure. It is demonstrated that the cerebral blood flow was maintained regardless of whether blood pressure was decreased by cilnidipine. Furthermore, cilnidipine had the activity to shift downward the lower limit of autoregulation for cerebral blood flow according to the results of the estimation of the lower limit of autoregulation for cerebral blood flow by exsanguination (Watanabe et al., 1995b). Interestingly, an antihypertensive and anti-sympathetic dose of cilnidipine reduced the size of cerebral infarction in the rat focal brain ischemia model in contrast to nilvadipine (Takahara et al., 2004), which is in accordance with previous study using a peptidic N-type Ca^{2+} channel blocker ω-conotoxin MVIIA. Thus, the results may support that N-type Ca^{2+} channel activation includes pathophysiological process of brain ischemia.

3.7 Metabolic syndrome

Pancreatic insulin secretion from β-cells and glucagon secretion from α-cells in the islets of Langerhans are Ca^{2+}-dependent processes initiated by Ca^{2+} influx probably through N-type Ca^{2+} channels. In a study using N-type Ca^{2+} channel α_{1B}-subunit-deficient homozygous knockout mice fed normal diet, there was improved glucose tolerance without any change in insulin sensitivity, and also body weight gain reduced in the mice fed a high-fat diet (Takahashi et al., 2005). In another study with fructose-fed rats, insulin sensitivity was significantly lower than in controls, and insulin resistance improved significantly after cilnidipine treatment (Takada et al., 2001). These imply that N-type Ca^{2+} channels play a significant role in glucose homeostasis.

Clinically, it was revealed that cilnidipine significantly reduced 24-hour urinary catecholamines in hypertensive patients with type 2 diabetes, and thereby may improve insulin resistance (Takeda et al., 1999). Also, it is demonstrated that with cilnidipine treatment in patients with obesity, fasting serum immunoreactive insulin (F-IRI) and insulin resistance index as assessed by homeostasis model assessment (HOMA-R) lowered, and serum dehydroepiandrosterone (DHEA) and serum DHEA-sulfate (DHEA-S) increased (Ueshiba & Miyachi, 2002).

4. Pleiotropic effects of cilnidipine

Renoprotective, neuroprotective and cardioprotective effects of cilnidipine have been demonstrated in clinical practice or animal examinations. It is noticed that cilnidipine may have pleiotropic effects besides N-type Ca^{2+} channel-blocking action.

4.1 Anti-oxidation

Dihydropiridine derivatives including nifedipine have been reported to act as lipophilic chain-breaking antioxidants; however, there are larger differences in their lipophilicity among dihydropyridines. Lipophilicity of cilnidipine is greater than that of amlodipine, which implies that cilnidipine itself can reduce oxidative stress independently in addition to its N-type Ca^{2+} channel blockade action.

Excess reactive oxygen species play an essential role in the development of a variety of renal diseases such as glomerulonephritis and tubulointerstitial nephritis. Indeed, in the kidney, cilnidipine significantly inhibited the increase in NADPH oxidase-derived superoxide production, whereas amlodipine had no effect on the activation of NADPH oxidase in the deoxycorticosterone acetate-salt rat (Toba et al., 2011). Also, cilnidipine elicits podocyte-protection and anti-proteinuric effect in SHR/ND mcr-cp rat model of spontaneous hypertension through the reduction of renal AngII level and a subsequent reduction in oxidative stress (Fan et al., 2010). N-type Ca^{2+} channels localized in podocyte have been shown to play an important role in angiotensin II-induced superoxide production, which may partly explain the renoprotective mechanisms of cilnidipine. Antiproteinuric effect of cilnidipine in the CARTER study (Fujita et al., 2007) is in part explained by its superior antioxidant activity.

In addition, cilnidipine shows neuroprotection in the model of oxidative stress-induced neurotoxicity using PC12 cells (Lee et al., 2009), which may partly explain the mechanisms of cilnidipine that reduced infarction volume in the rat focal brain ischemia model.

4.2 Suppression of renin-angiotensin-aldosterone system

It is widely known that renin secretion from the juxtaglomerular apparatus is closely associated with renal sympathetic nerve activity. Thus, cilnidipine may alter renin-angiotensin-aldosterone system. In recent studies using spontaneously hypertensive rats, whereas an L-type Ca^{2+} channel blocker amlodipine increased plasma renin activity and angiotensin II levels at antihypertensive doses, cilnidipine failed to affect plasma renin activity or plasma norepinephrine and angiotensin II levels, which strongly supports that cilnidipine suppresses renin-angiotensin system through sympathetic N-type Ca^{2+} channel blockade (Konda et al., 2009). In a previous study using the canine cardiac sudden death model, it was found for the first time that cilnidipine decreased the plasma concentration aldosterone level (Takahara et al., 2009). The curious action of cilnidipine was also confirmed in hypertensive rats. A recent study has clearly demonstrated that the endocrine mechanisms of angiotensin II-induced aldosterone production in the adrenocortical cells are closely associated with activities of N-type Ca^{2+} channels (Aritomi et al., 2011a).

Antihypertensive therapies with angiotensin II receptor blockers sometimes activate renin-angiotensin system. As shown in Fig. 3, increases in plasma renin activity and plasma angiotensin II levels can be observed by oral administration of valsartan in spontaneously hypertensive rats, which were effectively suppressed by cilnidipine but not by amlodipine (Aritomi et al., 2011b). Thus, cilnidipine is expected to provide synergistic and effective therapeutic strategies when administered with angiotensin II receptor blockers.

4.3 Abbreviation of prolonged QT-interval

The heart of canine chronic atrioventricular block model (cardiac sudden death model) is known to have a ventricular electrical remodeling, which mimics the pathophysiology of long QT syndrome (Sugiyama, 2008). Using this model, we explored a new pharmacological therapeutic strategy for prevention of cardiac sudden death (Fig. 4; Takahara et al., 2009). Amlodipine, cilnidipine or an angiotensin II receptor blocker candesartan was orally administered to the dogs for 4 weeks. Amlodipine and cilnidipine decreased the blood pressure, while candesartan hardly affected it. The QT interval and monophasic action potential duration were shortened only in the cilnidipine group, but such effects were not observed in the amlodipine or candesartan group. Plasma concentrations of angiotensin II

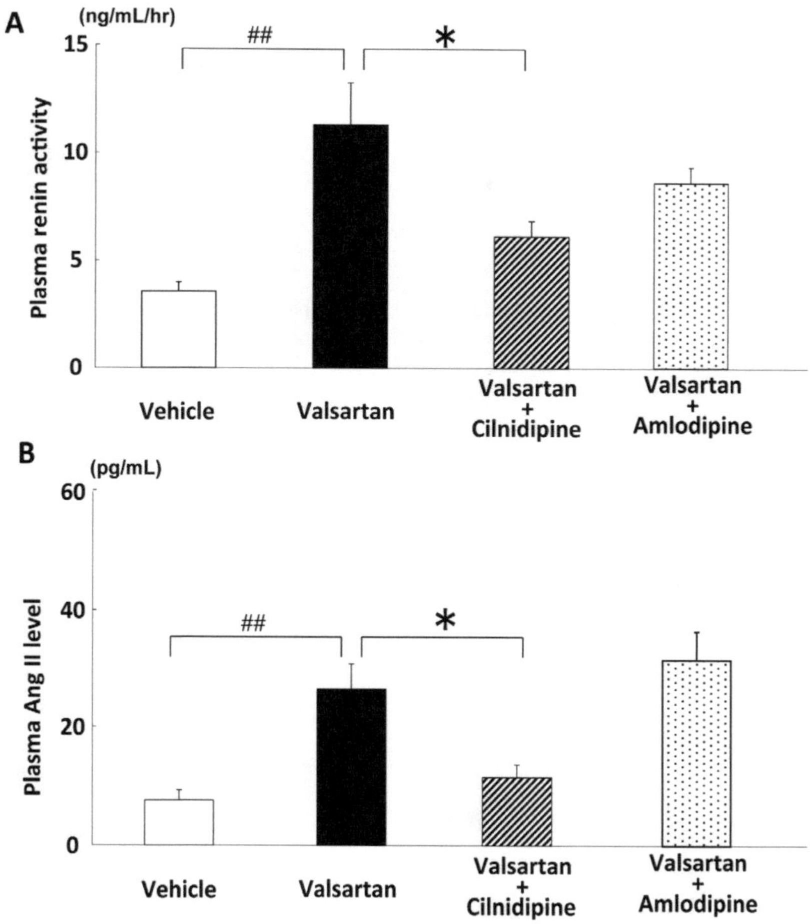

Fig. 3. Effects of combined administration of valsartan and amlodipine or cilnidipine on plasma renin activity (A) and plasma angiotensin II (Ang II) level (B) in spontaneously hypertensive rats. The oral doses of valsartan, amlodipine and cilnidipine were 10, 1 and 1 mg/kg, respectively. Values are expressed as means±SE. ##P < 0.01, vehicle vs. valsartan alone, *P < 0.05, Ca^{2+} channel blockers plus valsartan vs. valsartan alone. Data are quoted and modified from Aritomi et al., 2011b.

and aldosterone decreased in the cilnidipine group. On the other hand, elevation of plasma concentrations of angiotensin II and aldosterone was detected in the amlodipine group. Cilnidipine is expected to restore similar electrical remodeling process to pathophysiology of chronic atrioventricular block. Indeed, a recent electrophysiological study has demonstrated that some cardiac K^+ channels (I_{Ks} and I_{to}) are downregulated in the diabetic canine heart, leading to QT interval prolongation. Long QT interval has also been reported in patients with various cardiovascular diseases including hypertension with hypertrophy, hypertrophic cardiomyopathy and end-stage renal failure (Takahara et al., 2009). Therefore, long-term blockade of L/N-type Ca^{2+} channels may ameliorate the ventricular electrical remodeling in the hypertrophied heart leading to QT-interval prolongation, which will provide a novel therapeutic strategy.

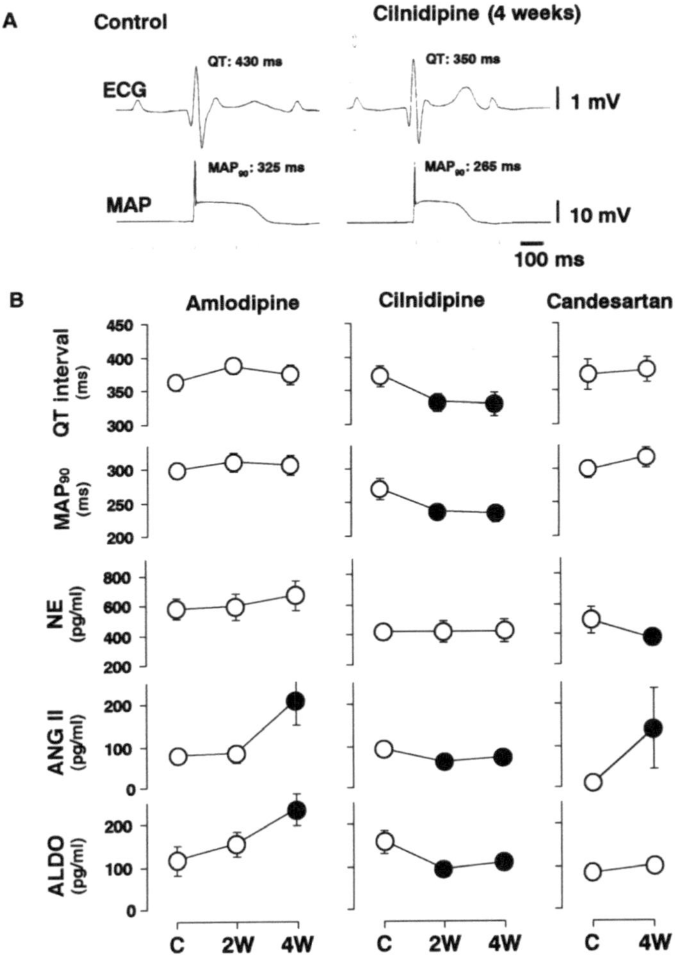

Fig. 4. Effects on electrocardiogram (ECG) and monophasic action potential (MAP) signal during idioventricular rhythm in chronic atrioventricular block dogs. A: Typical tracings of effects of cilnidipine on ECG and MAP signal. B: Effects of amlodipine (2.5mg/day), cilnidipine (5mg/day) and candesartan (12mg/day) on QT interval, MAP duration and plasma levels of norepinephrine (NE), angiotensin II (ANG II) and aldosterone (ALDO). These parameters were obtained at pre-drug control (C) and 2 weeks (2W) and 4 weeks (4W) after the start of drug daily administration. Data are presented as the means±SE. Closed symbols represent the significant differences from each pre-drug control (C) value by $p<0.05$. Data are quoted and modified from Takahara et al., 2009.

5. Conclusion

Cilnidipine is a promising Ca^{2+} channel blocker as the 4th generation with a rational pharmacological profile; i.e. dual L/N-type Ca^{2+} channel-blocking action. The blockade of N-type Ca^{2+} channels effectively suppresses neurohumoral regulation in the cardiovascular system, including sympathetic nervous system and renin-angiotensin-aldosterone system. Thus, cilnidipine is expected to be favorable for various types of complication of hypertension. Indeed, its advantage is demonstrated by the clinical study showing that cilnidipine is superior to amlodipine in preventing the progression of proteinuria in patients with hypertension and chronic renal disease (Fujita et al., 2007). The currently described information suggests that cilnidipine is a new type of antihypertensive drug distinguished from other L-type Ca^{2+} channel blockers or even other antihypertensives, which will be useful for selection of antihypertensive drugs according to the pathophysiological condition of a patient.

6. References

Aritomi, S.; Koganei, H.; Wagatsuma, H.; Mitsui, A.; Ogawa, T.; Nitta, K. & Konda, T. (2010). The N-type and L-type calcium channel blocker cilnidipine suppresses renal injury in Dahl rats fed a high-salt diet. *Heart and Vessels*, Vol 25, No.6, (November 2010), pp.549-555, ISSN 0910-8327.

Aritomi, S.; Wagatsuma, H.; Numata, T.; Uriu, Y.; Nogi, Y.; Mitsui, A.; Konda, T.; Mori, Y. & Yoshimura, M. (2011a). Expression of N-type calcium channels in human adrenocortical cells and their contribution to corticosteroid synthesis. *Hypertension Research*, Vol.34, No.2, (February 2011), pp. 193-201, ISSN 0916-9636.

Aritomi, S.; Niinuma, T.; Ogawa, T.; Konda, T. & Nitta, K. (2011b). Effect of an N-type calcium antagonist on angiotensin II-renin feedback. *American Journal of Nephrology*, Vol.33, No.2, (February 2011), pp. 168-175, ISSN 0250-8095.

Catterall, WA.; Striessnig, J.; Snutch, TP. & Perez-Reyes, E. (2003). International Union of Pharmacology. XL. Compendium of voltage-gated ion channels: calcium channels. *Pharmacological Reviews*, Vol.55, No.4, (December 2003), pp. 579-581, ISSN 0031-6997.

Fan, YY.; Kohno, M.; Nakano, D.; Ohsaki, H.; Kobori, H.; Suwarni, D.; Ohashi, N.; Hitomi, H.; Asanuma, K.; Noma, T.; Tomino, Y.; Fujita, T. & Nishiyama, A. (2010). Cilnidipine suppresses podocyte injury and proteinuria in metabolic syndrome rats: possible involvement of N-type calcium channel in podocyte. *Journal of Hypertension*, Vol.28, No.5, (May 2010), pp. 1034-1043, ISSN 0263-6352.

Fan, L.; Yang, Q.; Xiao, XQ.; Grove, KL.; Huang, Y.; Chen, ZW.; Furnary, A. & He, GW. (2011). Dual actions of cilnidipine in human internal thoracic artery: inhibition of calcium channels and enhancement of endothelial nitric oxide synthase. *Journal of Thoracic and Cardiovascular Surgery*, Vol.141, No.4, (April 2011), pp. 1063-1069, ISSN 0022- 5223.

Fujita, T.; Ando, K.; Nishimura, H.; Ideura, T.; Yasuda, G.; Isshiki, M. & Takahashi, K. Cilnidipine versus Amlodipine Randomised Trial for Evaluation in Renal Disease (CARTER) Study Investigators. (2007). Antiproteinuric effect of the calcium channel blocker cilnidipine added to renin-angiotensin inhibition in hypertensive patients with chronic renal disease. *Kidney International*, Vol.72, No.12, (December 2007), pp. 1543-1549, ISSN 0085-2538.

Hirning, LD.; Fox, AP.; McCleskey, EW.; Olivera, BM.; Thayer, SA.; Miller, RJ. & Tsien, RW. (1988). Dominant role of N-type Ca^{2+} channels in evoked release of norepinephrine from sympathetic neurons. *Science*, Vol.239, No.4835, (January 1988), pp. 57-61, ISSN 0036-8075.

Ishizaka, T.; Takahara, A.; Iwasaki, H.; Mitsumori, Y.; Kise, H.; Nakamura, Y. & Sugiyama, A. (2010). Cardiovascular effects of azelnidipine in comparison with those of amlodipine assessed in the halothane-anaesthetized dog. *Basic & Clinical Pharmacology & Toxicology*, Vol.106, No.2, (February 2010), pp. 135-143, ISSN 1742-7835.

Kimura, T.; Takeuchi, A. & Satoh, S. (1994). Inhibition by ω-conotoxin GVIA of adrenal catecholamine release in response to endogenous and exogenous acetylcholine. *European Journal of Pharmacology*, Vol.264, No.2, (October 1994), pp. 169-175, ISSN 0014-2999.

Konda, T.; Takahara, A.; Maeda, K.; Dohmoto, H. & Yoshimoto, R. (2001). Effects of a dual L/N-type Ca^{2+} channel blocker cilnidipine on neurally mediated chronotropic response in anesthetized dogs. *European Journal of Pharmacology*, Vol.413, No.1, (February 2001), pp. 117-120, ISSN 0014-2999.

Konda, T.; Enomoto, A.; Aritomi, S.; Niinuma, K.; Koganei, H.; Ogawa, T. & Nitta, K. (2009). Different effects of L/N-type and L-type calcium channel blockers on the renin-angiotensin-aldosterone system in SHR/Izm. *American Journal of Nephrology*, Vol.30, No.2, (August 2009), pp. 155-161, ISSN 0250-8095.

Konno, Y. & Kimura, K. (2008). Vasodilatory effect of cilnidipine, an L-type and N-type calcium channel blocker, on rat kidney glomerular arterioles. *International Heart Journal*, Vol.49, No.6, (November 2008), pp. 723-732, ISSN 1349-2365.

Kosaka, T.; Nakagawa, M.; Ishida, M.; Iino, K.; Watanabe, H.; Hasegawa, H. & Ito, H. (2009). Cardioprotective effect of an L/N-type calcium channel blocker in patients with hypertensive heart disease. *Journal of Cardiology*, Vol.54, No.2, (October 2009), pp. 262-272, ISSN 0914-5087.

Lee, YJ.; Park, KH.; Park, HH.; Kim, YJ.; Lee, KY.; Kim ,SH. & Koh, SH. (2009). Cilnidipine mediates a neuroprotective effect by scavenging free radicals and activating the phosphatidylinositol 3-kinase pathway. *Journal of Neurochemistry*, Vol.111, No.1, (October 2009), pp. 90-100, ISSN 0022-3042.

Nagai, H.; Minatoguchi, S.; Chen, XH.; Wang, N.; Arai, M.; Uno, Y.; Lu, C.; Misao, Y.; Onogi, H.; Kobayashi, H.; Takemura, G.; Maruyama, R.; Fujiwara, T. & Fujiwara, H. (2005). Cilnidipine, an N+L-type dihydropyridine Ca channel blocker, suppresses the occurrence of ischemia/reperfusion arrhythmia in a rabbit model of myocardial infarction. *Hypertension Research*, Vol.28, No.4, (April 2005), pp. 361-368, ISSN 0916-9636.

Ogasawara, A.; Hisa, H. & Satoh, S. (1993). An intracellular calcium release inhibitor TMB-8 suppresses renal nerve stimulation-induced antinatriuresis in dogs. *Journal of Pharmacology and Experimental Therapeutics*, Vol.264, No.1, (January 1993), pp. 117-121, ISSN 0022-3565.

Saitoh, M.; Sugiyama, A.; Nakamura, Y. & Hashimoto, K. (2003). Antianginal effects of L-type and N- type calcium channel blocker cilnidipine assessed using the vasopressin-induced experimental angina model of rats. *Journal of Pharmacological Sciences*, Vol.91, Supplement I, (March 2003), pp. 152P, ISSN 1347-8613.

Sugiyama, A. (2008). Sensitive and reliable proarrhythmia in vivo animal models for predicting drug-induced torsades de pointes in patients with remodelled hearts. *British Journal of Pharmacology*, Vol.154, No.7, (August 2008), pp. 1528-1537, ISSN 0007-1188.

Taira, N. (1987). Differences in cardiovascular profile among calcium antagonists. *American Journal of Cardiology*, Vol.59, No.3, (January 1987), pp. 24B–29B, ISSN 0002-9149.

Takahara, A. (2009). Cilnidipine: a new generation Ca^{2+} channel blocker with inhibitory action on sympathetic neurotransmitter release. *Cardiovascular Therapeutics*, Vol.27, No.2, (Summer 2009), pp. 124-39, ISSN 1755-5914.

Takahara, A.; Dohmoto, H.; Hisa, H.; Satoh, S. & Yoshimoto, R. (1997). Cilnidipine attenuates renal nerve stimulation-induced renal vasoconstriction and antinatriuresis in anesthetized dogs. *Japanese Journal of Pharmacology*, Vol.75, No.1, (September 1997), pp. 27-32, ISSN 1347-8613.

Takahara, A.; Koganei, H.; Takeda, T. & Iwata, S. (2002). Antisympathetic and hemodynamic property of a dual L/N-type Ca^{2+} channel blocker cilnidipine in rats. *European Journal of Pharmacology*, Vol.434, No.1-2, (January 2002) pp. 43–47, ISSN 0014-2999.

Takahara, A.; Konda, T.; Enomoto, A. & Kondo, N. (2004). Neuroprotective effects of a dual L/N-type Ca^{2+} channel blocker cilnidipine in the rat focal brain ischemia model. *Biological & Pharmaceutical Bulletin*, Vol.27, No.9, (September 2004), pp. 1388–1391, ISSN 0918-6158.

Takahara, A.; Iwasaki, H.; Nakamura, Y. & Sugiyama, A. (2007). Cardiac effects of L/N-type Ca^{2+} channel blocker cilnidipine in anesthetized dogs. *European Journal of Pharmacology*, Vol.565, No.1-3, (June 2007), pp. 166-70, ISSN 0014-2999.

Takahara, A.; Nakamura, Y.; Wagatsuma, H.; Aritomi, S.; Nakayama, A.; Satoh, Y.; Akie, Y. & Sugiyama, A. (2009). Long-term blockade of L/N-type Ca^{2+} channels by cilnidipine ameliorates repolarization abnormality of the canine hypertrophied heart. *British Journal of Pharmacology*, Vol.158, No.5, (November 2009), pp. 1366-1374, ISSN 0007-1188.

Takahashi, E.; Ito, M.; Miyamoto, N.; Nagasu, T.; Ino, M. & Tanaka, I. (2005). Increased glucose tolerance in N-type Ca^{2+} channel α_{1B}-subunit gene-deficient mice. *International Journal of Molecular Medicine*, Vol.15, No.6, (June 2005), pp. 937–944, ISSN 1107-3756.

Takada, M.; Ura, N.; Higashiura, K.; Murakami, H.; Togashi, N. & Shimamoto, K. (2001). Effects of cilnidipine on muscle fiber composition, capillary density and muscle blood flow in fructose-fed rats. *Hypertension Research*, Vol.24, No.5, (April 2001), pp. 565-572, ISSN 0916-9636.

Takeda, S.; Ueshiba, H.; Hattori, Y. & Irie, M. (1999). Cilnidipine, the N- and L-type calcium channel antagonist, reduced on 24-h urinary catecholamines and C-peptide in hypertensive non-insulin-dependent diabetes mellitus. *Diabetes Research and Clinical Practice*, Vol.44, No.3, (June 1999), pp. 197-205, ISSN 0168-8227.

Tanaka, H. & Shigenobu, K. (2005). Pathophysiological significance of T-type Ca^{2+} channels: T-type Ca^{2+} channels and drug development. *Journal of Pharmacological Sciences*, Vol.99, No.3, (November 2005), pp. 214-220, ISSN 1347-8613.

Toba, H.; Yoshida, M.; Tojo, C.; Nakano, A.; Oshima, Y.; Kojima, Y.; Noda, K.; Wang, J.; Kobara, M. & Nakata, T. (2011). L/N-type calcium channel blocker cilnidipine ameliorates proteinuria and inhibits the renal renin-angiotensin-aldosterone system in deoxycorticosterone acetate-salt hypertensive rats. *Hypertension Research*, Vol.34, No.4, (April 2011), pp. 521-529, ISSN 0916-9636.

Ueshiba, H. & Miyachi, Y. (2002). Effects of cilnidipine on adrenocortical steroid hormones and insulin resistance in hypertensive patients with obesity. *Therapeutic Research*, Vol.23, No.12, (December 2002), pp. 2493-2497, ISSN 0289-8020.

Uneyama, H.; Takahara, A.; Dohmoto, H.; Yoshimoto, R.; Inoue, K. & Akaike, N. (1997). Blockade of N-type Ca^{2+} current by cilnidipine (FRC-8653) in acutely dissociated rat sympathetic neurones. *British Journal of Pharmacology*, Vol.122, No.1, (September 1997), pp. 37–42, ISSN 0007-1188.

Uneyama, H.; Takahara, A.; Wakamori, M.; Mori, Y. & Yoshimoto, R. (1999a). Pharmacology of N-type Ca^{2+} channels distributed in cardiovascular system (Review). *International Journal of Molecular Medicine*, Vol.3, No.5, (May 1999), pp. 455-466, ISSN 1107-3756.

Uneyama, H.; Uchida, H.; Konda, T.; Yoshimoto, R. & Akaike, N. (1999b). Selectivity of dihydropyridines for cardiac L-type and sympathetic N-type Ca^{2+} channels. *European Journal of Pharmacology*, Vol.373, No.1, (May 1999), pp. 93–100, ISSN 0014-2999.

Varadi, G.; Mori, Y.; Mikala, G. & Schwartz, A. (1995). Molecular determinants of Ca^{2+} channel function and drug action. *Trends in Pharmacological Sciences*, Vol.16, No.2, (February 1995), pp. 43–49, ISSN 0165-6147.

Watanabe, K.; Hosono, M.; Dozen, M.; Kinoshita, A.; Arai, Y. & Hayashi, Y. (1995a). Inhibitory effect of cilnidipine (FRC-8653) on stroke and hypertensive lesions in stroke-prone spontaneously hypertensive rats. *Japanese Pharmacology & Therapeutics*, Vol.23, No.11, (November 1995), pp. 3013-3019, ISSN 0386-3603.

Watanabe, K.; Dozen, M. & Hayashi, Y. (1995b). Effect of cilnidipine (FRC-8653) on autoregulation of cerebral blood flow. *Folia Pharmacologica Japonica*, Vol.106, No.6, (December 1995), pp. 393-399, ISSN 0015-5691.

Yamagishi, T. Beneficial effect of cilnidipine on morning hypertension and white-coat effect in patients with essential hypertension. *Hypertension Research*, Vol.29, No.5, (May 2006), pp. 339-344, ISSN 0916-9636.

3

Hypertension and Chronic Kidney Disease: Cause and Consequence – Therapeutic Considerations

Elsa Morgado and Pedro Leão Neves
Nephrology Department, Hospital of Faro, Portugal

1. Introduction

There is a strong relationship between hypertension and Chronic Kidney Disease (CKD). Hypertension is an important cause of End-Stage Renal Disease (ESRD), contributing to the disease itself or, most commonly, contributing to its progression. On the other hand, hypertension is highly prevalent in CKD patients, playing a role in the high cardiovascular morbidity and mortality of this particular population. This chapter will focus on the pathogenesis of hypertension-related CKD and its role on the progression of renal disease itself. The pathogenesis and treatment of hypertension resulting from CKD will also be addressed.

2. Hypertension as a cause of CKD

The relationship between abnormal blood pressure and kidney dysfunction was first established in the 19th century. The prevalence of both, and of the associated burden of cardiovascular morbidity and mortality, has been dramatically increasing worldwide (Kearney et al., 2005; Kearney et al., 2004; Ong et al., 2007; Schoenborn & Heyman, 2009; USRDS 2010; Meguid El Nahas & Bello, 2005). Data from several renal databases identifies systemic hypertension as the second most common cause of ESRD, with Diabetes mellitus being the first. In the United States (US), hypertension is the leading cause of ESRD in African-American patients (USRDS 2010; Klag et al., 1996; Hsu et al., 2005). Additionally, for any given cause of CKD, the elevation in systemic blood pressure accelerates the rate at which the glomerular filtration rate (GFR) declines (Perry et al., 1995). This is particularly true for patients with proteinuric nephropathies (Jafar et al., 2003).

2.1 Pathogenesis of hypertensive renal damage

The exact mechanisms of kidney damage in patients with hypertension still remain elusive. Two complementary pathogenic mechanisms ultimately ending in kidney fibrosis and scarring have been proposed. One starts with the changes in systemic and renal macro and microvasculature leading to the loss of renal auto-regulation with elevation of intraglomerular capillary pressure and the consequent hyperfiltration-mediated injury.

Hyperfiltration leads to transglomerular loss of proteins which promotes the release of cytokines and growth factors by mesangial cells and downstream tubular epithelial cells. The second mechanism proposes endothelial dysfunction and loss of endogenous vasodilators as precipitating factors of hypoxic-ischemic injury. The consequent activation of the intrarrenal Renin Angiotensin System (RAS) and the increased release of cytokines and growth factors with recruitment of inflammatory cells stimulate apoptosis causing loss of normal kidney cells and increased matrix production, finally leading to progressive glomerular and interstitial fibrosis and scarring.

Evidence to support, this apparently straightforward, chain of events starting in systemic hypertension and culminating in ESRD, has been accumulating since the beginnings of the 20th century when Goldblatt conducted his first experiments in dogs driven hypertensive by the clipping of one renal artery: the two-kidney one clip model of hypertension (Goldblatt, 1964). The brilliancy of this model rests on the existence of a control organ: the clipped kidney was protected from the deleterious effects of blood pressure. In fact, vascular damage was not found in the clipped kidneys. More recently, other authors reported that the clipped kidney is also protected from the effects of immunological mediators (Wenzel et al., 2002).

Extension of this model to rats and rabbits confirmed Goldblatt findings (Eng et al., 1994; Wenzel et al., 2002). These later experiments also documented the pivotal role of changes in renal macro and microvasculature to induce and maintain a vicious cycle, where hypertension causes vascular lesions which in turn will further increase blood pressure, even after its primary cause has been removed (Rettig et al., 1990).

Further investigation on animal models, as well as on genetic models of hypertension, allowed the description of three different stages of preglomerular vascular change. The histopathological resemblance between these experimentally induced vascular lesions and those observed in benign and malignant nephrosclerosis in human kidneys have long been documented. Medial thickening with narrowing of the lumen resulting from hypertrophy of smooth muscle cells (Nordborg et al., 1983; Hampton et al., 1989; Vial & Boyd 1989; Lee, 1987; Mulvany & Aalkjaar 1990; Owens & Schartz, 1982; Chobanian et al., 1984; Ross, 1993) is followed by segmental hyalinosis of the vessel wall of interlobular arteries and afferent arterioles. In humans studies using light microscopy and imunofluorescence these lesions were better characterized and termed "benign nephrosclerosis" (Valenzuela, 1980; Fisher,1966). Finally, the most severe type of hypertensive renal vascular lesion, similar to "malignant nephrosclerosis", is proliferation of the intima resulting in the typical onion-like appearance and extremely narrow vessels predominantly affecting the interlobular arteries and afferent arterioles (Klemperer & Otani, 1931). The previous existence of medial hypertrophy and, or, increased collagen content in the arterial wall were pre-requisites for the development of this final stage (Helmchen et al., 1984, Bidani et al., 1994). However, in humans even the early lesions of malignant nephrosclerosis affect the intima (Ellis, 1942; Heptinstal, 1953; Somers, 1958).

After this initial chain of events, increased glomerular perfusion and elevation of glomerular capillary pressure resulting in hyperfiltration, lead to further damage of the affected glomerulus (Brenner, 1985; Klahr et al., 1988) and to increased filtration of proteins to the tubular lumen. Enhanced tubular reabsorption induces the synthesis of inflammatory and fibrotic factors, resulting in tubulointerstial ischemia, inflammation, up-regulation of oxidative stress and epithelial-to-mesenchimal transdifferentiation eventually culminating in fibrosis (Ruggenenti & Remuzzi, 2000; Mayer et al., 1993; Abbate et al., 1998; Fine et al., 1998; Sánchez-Lozada et al., 2003; Higgins et al., 2007; Tian et al., 2008; Leh et al., 2011; Dussaule et al., 2011). The involvement of inflammation in the progression of CKD was widely demonstrated in experimental models of non-imunologic kidney disease (Bottinger & Bitzer, 2002; Müller, 2000, 2001; Fujihara, 1998, 2000; Romero et al., 1999; Mazzali et al., 2001; Eddy & Giachelli, 1995; Largo et al., 1999; Gómez-Garre et al., 2001; Zoja et al., 1998; Takase et al., 2003; Alvarez et al., 2002).

Traditionally, the glomeruli have been in the centre of attention particularly in view of the hyperfiltration hypothesis involving the degradation and sclerosis of the remaining nephrons. However, the notion that tubulointerstitial fibrosis might rather cause than result from decreased glomerular function has gained strong evidence (Ong & Fine, 1994; Luft & Haller, 1995). Tubulointerstitial proliferation with incoming of inflammatory monocytes and macrophages, resulting from mechanical damage to the postglomerular interstitial vasculature, were also described, establishing the tubules and the interstitium as additional sites of early hypertensive damage (Eng et al., 1994). Furthermore, the up-regulation of the intrarrenal RAS, hypothetically mediated by local ischemia, is associated with increased expression of Angiotensin Converting Enzyme (ACE) in proximal tubules and peri-tubular interstitium. Here, ACE can cleave angiotensinogen and bradykinins creating an imbalance in favor of the former with the consequent stimulation of proliferation, fibrosis and salt retention (Carlos & Jeanneret, 2003).

2.2 Epidemiology of hypertensive nephrosclerosis

The general term "nephrosclerosis", both benign and malignant, has been used to describe these lesions since the beginning of the 20th century. The causal relationship between malignant hypertension with fibrinoid necrosis and renal failure is consensual. On the other hand, the evidence for a relationship between milder degrees of hypertension and either benign nephrosclerosis and ESRD remains controversial (Zucchelli & Zuccala, 1995; Freedman et al., 1995; Kincaid-Smith, 1999).

In the past 30 years, at the start of dialysis, an increasing number of patients have been labeled as having hypertension-related ESRD (USRDS 2003). Although, only few of them have undergone a kidney biopsy (Weisstuch & Dworkin, 1992) making it impossible to exclude other causes of ESRD, such as atheroembolic disease, ischemic nephropathy secondary to atheromatous disease, or glomerulonephritis (Zucchelli & Zuccala, 1998; Freedman et al., 1995). On the other hand, the increased life expectancy of the general population, due to better anti-hypertensive control and better survival from cardiovascular events, providing a longer time for hypertensive renal disease to progress, could in fact account for this increased prevalence (Caetano et al., 1999). The MRFIT study established a consistent relationship between increasing levels of systolic and diastolic blood pressure and ESRD that was independent of several other relevant variables. Nevertheless, several other literature reports originating in studies conducted in the US and in the United Kingdom concluded that benign nephrosclerosis did not significantly progress to ESRD (Tomson et al., 1999; Kincaid-Smith, 1982, 1999). However, the exception was provided by Africa-American patients in whom a higher risk of progression to ESRD was widely demonstrated in all age groups (Rostand, 1982; Fogo, 1997; Marcantoni et al., 2002). This disproportion could not be explained by the higher prevalence and greater severity of hypertension in African-American patients or by socioeconomic determinants (Freedman 1993, 1995). Furthermore, in African-American patients progression for ESRD is faster across all levels of blood pressure (Klag et al., 1997; Shulman et al., 1989). Biopsy-proven hypertensive nephrosclerosis occurs earlier and is more severe in African-American than in Caucasian patients independently of blood presure values and proteinuria (Tracy et al., 1991; Perneger et al., 1995; Marcantoni et al., 2002). Traditionally, this excess of kidney damage has been associated with genetically or environmentally induced impairment of renal auto-regulation and amplification of profibrotic mechanisms (Campese et al., 1991; Duru et al., 1994; Suthanthiran et al., 1998).

Early studies from animal models with Dahl salt-sensitive rats, Spontaneous Hypertensive Rats, Fawn-hooded rats and Brown and Norway rats as well as the results of the AASKD trial suggested a genetic susceptibility to hypertensive vascular damage (Brown et al., 1996; Churchill et al., 1997; Freedman et al., 1998; Zarif et al., 2000; Agodoa et al., 2001). Several genetic alterations have been associated to a more rapid decline of renal function in African-American patients with hypertensive nephrosclerosis. Polymorphisms of the kallikrein (KLK1) gene promoter were associated with a higher risk of ESRD in the presence of hypertension in a population of African-American patients (Yu et al., 2002). Different genetic polymorphisms of the RAS have been linked to a greater progression to ESRD across a wide spectrum of populations and causes of CKD (Wong et al., 2008). Polymorphisms of TGF-β have also been implicated in hypertension and progressive fibrosis (August et al., 2000). Non-muscle myosin heavy chain 9 gene (MYH9) polymorphisms, leading to disruption of normal podocyte function, brought attention to the role of podocyte injury as a mechanism of kidney damage in hypertensive glomerulosclerosis (Freedman et al., 2009). Genetic variation within the loci of the adrenergic beta-1 receptor (ADRB1) gene is associated with increased adrenergic activity and an increased risk of progressive renal disease (Fung et al., 2009). Specific polymorphisms in the C - reactive protein gene predicted a higher risk for CKD progression, resistant to the action of ACE inhibitors in African-American patients (Hung et al., 2010). Finally, mutations in the human methylenetetrahydrofolate reductase (MTHFR) gene were associated with elevated levels of homocysteine and a faster decline of renal function over time in African-American patients (Fung et al., 2011). Very recently a study, conducted in a population of Hispanic descent reported an association between polymorphisms of vascular endothelial growth factor (VEGF) and hypertensive nephropathy with subsequent progression to ESRD (Yang et al., 2011).

3. Pathogenesis of hypertension in chronic kidney disease

Although the kidney is also involved in essential or primary hypertension, its insufficiency causes high BLOOD PRESSURE, contributing to 2-5 % of all cases of hypertension or half the cases of all forms of secondary hypertension (Kaplan, 2006b). The pathogenesis of hypertension-related to CKD is complex and multifactorial, mainly in the late stages of the renal disease. In addition to the classical factors, such as increased intravascular volume and excessive activity of the RAS, there are new recognized players such as increased activity of the sympathetic nervous system, endothelial dysfunction and alterations of several humoral and neural factors that promote an increase of the blood pressure. Hypertension is highly prevalent in CKD, being related with the level of renal function, the etiology of the kidney disease and the age of the patient. Patients with vascular disease, diabetes and polycystic kidney disease (PKD) are more prone to be hypertensive (Ridao et al., 2001). It is also known that as renal function worsens the prevalence of hypertension increases. Therefore, more than 80 % of the patients beginning renal replacement therapy have high blood pressure (Ridao et al., 2001, USRDS, 2010).

3.1 Sodium and volume status

The fundamental role of the kidney in the control of sodium and volume homeostasis is well acknowledged since the seminal studies of Dahl and Guyton. During the last decades, a bulk of evidence shows that volume expansion is the first and major pathogenic mechanism for hypertension in CKD. In the early stages of CKD, patients have already an increased exchangeable sodium and blood volume, which are correlated with the blood pressure level (Beretta-Piccoli et al, 1976).

According to the Guyton's whole-body auto-regulation concept, many organs, including the kidney and the brain, have the ability to maintain a relatively constant blood flow in the presence of variations of the perfusion pressure (Coleman & Guyton, 1969). Guyton proposed that this auto-regulation could be responsible for the secondary increase of the peripheral resistance in the presence of blood volume expansion, as it occurs in CKD (Guyton et al, 1980). Therefore, initially, an augment of the blood volume increases the cardiac output and simultaneously the peripheral vascular resistance fell. Later, the auto-regulatory increase of the vascular resistance causes a pressure natriuresis (Navar, & Majid, 1996), with normalization of the cardiac output and maintenance of high blood pressure values.

3.2 The Renin-Angiotensin System

The relevance of the RAS, in physiological terms, is based on its capacity to regulate arterial pressure and sodium balance. When the blood pressure or perfusion fall, or the sympathetic activity increases, the juxtaglomerular cells secrete renin, which cleaves angiotensinogen, leading to an increase in angiotensin II (AII) levels. This octapeptide is a powerful vasoconstrictor and stimulates the production of aldosterone, which, in turn, increases renal sodium reabsorption, and closes the regulatory feedback loop. However, if the blood volume is normal, the increased activity of the RAS produces an abnormal rise in the blood pressure.

Only a small proportion of CKD patients have a measurable increase of the RAS (Acosta, 1982). However, this activity in most of these patients is inappropriately high in the volume-expanded milieu of CKD (Davies et al, 1973; Mailloux, 2001). Furthermore, in CKD, mainly secondary to vascular disease, diabetes or PKD, in areas of renal injury or ischemia there is a greater production of local and intra-renal AII which then exacerbates systemic hypertension (Acosta, 1982;Rosenberg et al, 1994).

3.3 Oxidative stress and nitric oxide antagonism

"Oxidative stress is an imbalance between oxidants and anti-oxidants in favor of the oxidants, potentially leading to damage"(Sies, 1997). In CKD there is an excess of oxidant molecules such as superoxide and hydrogen peroxide and a decrease of anti-oxidant ones, such as catalase, superoxide dismutase and glutathione dismutase (Vaziri et al., 2002). The excess of reactive oxygen species may directly stimulate vascular contraction or reduce nitric oxide, contributing to hypertension in CKD (Hu et al., 1998). In addition, it is known that anti-oxidant agents can reduce the blood pressure in animal models of hypertension (Vaziri et al., 1997). The endothelial-derived nitric oxide has the capacity to maintain the vascular tone and to produce vasodilatation, through the activation of guanylate cyclase. In CKD, there is an increase of asymmetric dimethylarginine, an inhibitor of nitric oxide synthase (Leone et al., 1992). Moreover, has we pointed out before, the increase amount of reactive oxygen species in CKD impair nitric oxide effects. These two factors are responsible for a decrease nitric oxide activity in CKD which contribute to endothelial dysfunction and increased blood pressure.

3.4 Sympathetic Nervous System and Renal Dopaminergic System

The Sympathetic Nervous System activity is increased in CKD, as was demonstrated almost 20 years ago (Converse et al., 1992). Afferent signals from the diseased kidney are transmitted to the vasomotor control center in the brain increasing the blood pressure (Rump et al, 2000). In addition, increased plasma noradrenaline levels are often high in CKD patients. Evidence for the role of sympathetic nervous system is provided by the fall of blood pressure after renal sympathetic denervation or after bilateral nephrectomy (Khawaja et al, 2011).

Dopamine, a precursor of noradrenaline, has a natriuretic effect by inhibiting Na-K-ATPase in proximal tubular segments. Patients with CKD have reduced urinary excretion of dopamine (Casson et al, 1983) and decreased activity of the renal dopaminergic system, which correlates well with the degree of renal dysfunction (Pestana et al, 2001). These data show that the reduced activity of renal dopaminergic system in CKD, by decreasing the sodium excretion, may be another factor connected with the hypertension of CKD.

3.5 Miscellaneous

Endothelin is a family of four 21 amino acid peptides and ET-1, the predominant isoform, is produced by endothelial cells. It can mediate vasoconstriction when binds to its A and B receptors in vascular smooth muscle cells. Vasodilation results from the interaction with the B receptor in endothelial cells. In CKD, endothelin levels are increased and the use of selective endothelin A receptor antagonist produces reduction of blood pressure associated with renal vasodilatation (Goddard et al, 2004).

Parathormone starts to rise early in CKD. Its role in the pathogenesis of hypertension remains controversial. It has been shown, by some but not all authors that the parathormone can increase intracellular calcium and aggravate hypertension and that parathyroidectomy may improve blood pressure control.

The role of Endogenous Digitalis-like Factors (EDLFs) in sodium or volume dependent hypertension was elucidated only recently, after several decades of intense research. The EDLFs include quite a few substances, produced in the adrenal gland or in the hypothalamus, that inhibit the Na-K-ATPase in cell membranes, being at the same time natriuretic and vasoconstrictors (Takahashi et al, 2011). The high levels of EDLFs in CKD

(Hamlyn et al, 1996; Komiyama et al, 2005), secondary to an increased sodium content and expanded blood volume, may also contribute to the hypertension commonly seen in this population.

4. Considerations about hypertension treatment in CKD

The treatment of hypertension in CKD has three main goals: blood pressure control; delaying the progression of CKD itself; decreasing the risk of cardiovascular complications in this particular population. The role of non-drug therapy is frequently underestimated. However, salt restriction and lifestyle modifications are invaluable to achieve the goals defined above. Drug therapy is fundamental, and at later stages of CKD, double or multiple drug associations are often needed. RAS antagonists should the preferred drugs and their association with diuretics mandatory.

4.1 Salt restriction and life style modifications

Given that one of the main causes of CKD related hypertension is increased extracellular volume (or exchangeable sodium), dietary sodium restriction makes every sense. Excess dietary salt, typical of Western Countries, is clearly associated with the massive number of hypertensive patients in modern societies and, in the other extreme, it is well known that in primitive civilizations with low sodium intake, the prevalence of hypertension is irrelevant (Carvalho et al, 1989). Guidelines on CKD recommend a low sodium ingestion (70–100mmol/day) in patients with CKD (KDOQI, 2004; Joint Specialty Committee Guidelines, 2006; Levin et al, 2008). This suggestion is based on the evidence that a lower sodium intake is associated with a reduction of the blood pressure values (Sacks et al, 2001), increases the protective effect of ACE inhibitors in patients with proteinuria (Heeg et al, 1989) and, possibly, declines the progression of renal failure (Ciancaruso et al, 1998). Concerning life style changes, it is recommended to CKD patients to have a healthy life. Cigarette smoking, a well known cardiovascular risk factor also works as a renal risk factor. Smoking increases blood pressure by stimulating the sympathetic nervous system and also by rising plasma endothelin levels (Orth, 2003; Halimi & Mimran, 2000). The related excessive production of oxygen-free radicals can produce endothelial dysfunction and consequently be another factor implicated in the increase of blood pressure. It is critical to stop smoking, because this preventable risk factor can hasten the progression of chronic renal insufficiency in diabetic and non-diabetic nephropathies, independently of gender and race (Orth, 2003). Reduction of alcohol ingestion is also another useful decision, not because it is related with worsening of the renal function itself, but rather because it can be associated with smoking and obesity (Suter & Schutz, 2008). Weight loss in hypertensive obese patients is associated with reductions of the blood pressure, proteinuria and left ventricular hypertrophy, with benefits in terms of total cardiovascular outcomes. In CKD patients a favorable impact was also demonstrated: a decrease in proteinuria and better blood pressure control (Praga & Morales, 2006). Weight reduction may improve insulin resistance and decreases inflammation and oxidative stress beyond positive actions on the RAS and sympathetic nervous system. Furthermore, it may also slow down the progression to ESRD. The regular practice of exercise also has a beneficial effect on CKD patients. A high-quality exercise program can improve many indicators of physical performance, as well as all cardiovascular indices. Exercise may improve the control of blood pressure and endothelial function and decrease inflammation and insulin resistance (Johansen, 2007). Moreover, physical exercise has no untoward effect on progression of CKD. However, since this population has a potential bigger risk of musculoskeletal injuries and cardiac events it is mandatory to perform an accurate medical checkout before enrolling any exercise program.

4.2 Pharmacological therapy

The need to employ anti-hypertensive drugs mainly in the late stages of the disease is mandatory in almost all CKD patients. It is, often, necessary to use multiple drug regimens to control the blood pressure levels adequately and a constant evaluation of patient compliance and frequent medical reassessment meetings are required.

4.2.1 What should be the target blood pressure?

Nearly all guidelines concerning CKD patients support that blood pressure should be targeted to less than 130/80 mmHg (Chobanian et al, 2003; KDOQI, 2004; Levin et al, 2008). Despite major well designed randomized controlled trials (RCT) (Klahr et al, 1994; Estacio et al, 2000; Wright et al, 2002; Ruggenenti et al, 2005), there is no clear evidence that a blood pressure target < 130/80 mmHg is better, in terms of renal disease progression in CKD patients. A recently published systematic review did not show any advantage, regarding progression of CKD, in keeping blood pressure < 130/80 mmHg (Upadhyay et al, 2011). Post-hoc analysis of the MDRD and ABCD studies showed some benefits in the group of patients with a better control of the blood pressure, and two meta-analyses (Makki et al, 1995; Casas et al, 2005) also showed a protracted progression of the CKD in patients with lower blood pressure levels. Furthermore, another meta-analysis including 11 RCT with non-diabetic CKD patients, showed that those with systolic blood pressure between 110-119 mmHg, had the lowest risk of progression of CKD, and that this risk was greatly increased in patients with systolic blood pressure > 130 mmHg (Jafar et al, 2003). Finally, Appel and co-workers demonstrated that in African-American patients with CKD and proteinuria, intensive blood pressure treatment decreased the risk of progression of renal failure (Appel et al, 2010). Secondary analysis from large RCT with antagonists of the RAS, such as the HOPE, IDNT and ADVANCE studies, proved that hypertension treatment in CKD patients can reduce the risk of cardiovascular events (Mann et al, 2001; Pohl et al, 2005; Heerspink et al, 2010). However, insofar no RCT was able to prove that a blood pressure < 130/80 mmHg is better in terms of cardiovascular outcomes. On the other hand, it must be kept in mind that lowering the blood pressure < 120/70 mmHg, mainly in older patients, can increase the progression of renal failure (van Bemmel et al, 2006) and enhance the probability of a cardiovascular event (Pohl et al, 2005; Hirsh et al, 2008). In brief, there is no strong evidence to have a blood pressure target < 130/80 mmHg, and we should maintain the goal of blood pressure < 140/90 mmHg, mostly in the elderly. However, in patients under 60 years with proteinuria a lower target might be allowed.

4.2.2 Which anti-hypertensive drug must we choose?

We must choose a drug to control the blood pressure, with the ability to slow down the inexorable progression of CKD and decrease the cardiovascular risk of this population. Hypertension control, by itself, can delay the progression of CKD, as Mogensen reported more than 30 years ago, using diuretics and a Beta Blocker in type I diabetic patients with nephropathy (Mogensen, 1976). Notwithstanding, in the last decades, the superiority of the ACE inhibitors, and lately of the angiotensin receptor blockers (ARB), in terms of preventing the progression of CKD and also in terms of reducing cardiovascular morbidity and mortality have been widely reported in medical literature. The benefits of ACE inhibitors and ARB are far beyond and independent of blood pressure control. The mechanisms of renal protection result from hemodynamic and non-hemodynamic actions: decrease of intraglomerular hydrostatic pressure, decrease of protein excretion, and decrease of AII activity (Sica, 2003). This octapeptide is also a powerful cytokine with non-hemodynamic properties such as proinflammatory and profibrotic actions. AII upregulates the production of adhesion molecules, cytokines and chemokines, increasing the number of inflammatory cells in the kidney. It also stimulates extracellular matrix accumulation through the production of profibrotic factors, such as transforming growth factor-β. The decrease of AII activity observed with these drugs explains, in part, the extra advantages of their use in CKD patients. Several RCT and meta-analysis, in type 1 and 2 diabetic patients as well as in non-diabetic patients, confirmed that ACE inhibitors and ARB must be first choice drugs in renal patients, since they effectively slow the progression of CKD (Jafar et al, 2003; Lewis et al, 1993; Lewis et al, 2001; Brenner et al, 2001; Jafar et al, 2001). In addition, these particular drugs have the ability to reduce cardiovascular morbidity and mortality. In a post hoc analysis of the HOPE study, treatment with ramipril in patients with slight to moderate CKD decreased significantly the number of cardiovascular events (Mann et al, 2001). In the PEACE trial, trandolapril reduced the mortality in 27 % only in the subgroup of patients with renal insufficiency (Solomon et al, 2006) and in a recent meta-analysis, Balamuthusamy and co-workers found that RAS blockade in patients with non-diabetic renal disease was associated with a significant reduction in cardiovascular outcomes (Balamuthusamy et al, 2007). Concerning the secondary effects of these anti-hypertensive agents in renal patients, special attention must be given to: possible slight increase of the creatinine level (< 25 %), reflecting a decrease of the glomerular hyperfiltration, which means good news on the long run; a major increase of the creatinine level is suggestive of volume depletion (concomitant use of diuretics) or of bilateral renal artery stenosis; hyperkalemia is usually insignificant, but when severe it might be fatal; we must be aware of the potassium intake and of the use of other potentially hyperkalemic drugs, like aldosterone antagonists or non-steroid anti-inflammatory drugs; finally, we must also take into consideration that these drugs may also increase the need for higher dose of erythropoiesis stimulating agents (Neves et al, 2007).

4.2.3 Which drug association must we favor?

As stated previously, most patients will need two or more drugs to control hypertension and a stepwise approach should be pursued. After the prescription of an ACE inhibitor or an ARB, if there are no contra-indications, the choice of another anti-hypertensive agent must be dictated by any specific conditions of each patient. Diuretics are very useful and almost always mandatory, mainly in later stages of the disease, because of the presence of fluid overload. Thiazides can be used when the GFR > 30 ml/min/1,73 m^2 body surface area, being ineffective beyond this level. Then, we should rather use a loop diuretic such as indapamide or furosemide (KDOQI, 2004). Diuretics have the ability to diminish sodium reabsorption, thereby reversing hypervolemia and reducing the blood pressure. By reducing the blood volume and stimulating the renin activity, diuretics intensify the effect of ACE inhibitors and ARB. Potassium sparing agents must be avoided or used very carefully due to the risk of life threatening hyperkalemia, particularly if the patient is also under an ACE inhibitor or ARB (KDOQI, 2004). For all these reasons, in the CKD patient, diuretics should be the first class of anti-hypertensive drugs to be added to an ACE inhibitor or an ARB. Calcium Channel Blockers (CCB) are potent vasodilators and also have a relevant role in the control of the blood pressure in CKD patients. They are particularly indicated if the patient has angina or heart failure secondary to diastolic dysfunction (KDOQI, 2004). Due to distinct renal hemodynamic effects, the type CCB to use should not be indiscriminate. In fact, dihydropyridines by inhibiting the renal auto-regulatory capacity and by increasing the glomerular permeability, intensifying proteinuria (Nathan et al, 2005), are harmful in terms of CKD progression. This observation was well demonstrated in the AASK and IDNT trials (Wright et al, 2002, Lewis et al, 2001), where the dihydropyridine amlodipine was worse than the ACE inhibitor or the ARB regimen. However, the non-dihydropyridines, do not interfere with glomerular auto-regulation, and therefore do not exhibit deleterious effect in terms of proteinuria and renal function (Nathan et al, 2005; Bakris et al, 1996). In renal patients with proteinuria, the non-dihydropyridine CCB are a good choice to add to an ACE inhibitor to an ARB. On the contrary, they should be avoided in patients with second and third degree heart block or with congestive heart failure due to systolic dysfunction (KDOQI, 2004). Once the dihydropiridines have detrimental effects on renal function, it is recommended that they must be given in combination with kidney protecting drugs, such as the AII antagonists. In fact, in the ACCOMPLISH trial, the risk of progression of the CKD was lower in the group of patients treated with a combination of an ACE inhibitor with amlodipine than in the group treated with the ACE inhibitor and a diuretic (Bakris et al, 2010).. This study may support, at least in some patients, the use of a CCB as the first drug to add to an AII axis antagonist. It has been shown that this association may have a greater anti-inflammatory effect. Beta-Adrenergic Blockers comprise a heterogeneous group of drugs organized in classes according to their receptor selectivity, lipid-solubility, intrinsic sympathetic activity and membrane stabilizing capacity (Kaplan, 2006a). The use of a Beta-Adrenergic Blocker, in a renal patient, is almost always justified by the coexistence of ischemic heart disease. This class of drugs is specially indicated in patients with prior angina or myocardial infarction or with atrial tachycardia or fibrillation (KDOQI, 2004). The water soluble Beta-Adrenergic Blockers (atenolol, sotalol) are excreted by the kidney and may accumulate in CKD; the lipid soluble ones (propranolol, metoprolol) are metabolized in the liver and may be associated with central nervous system side effects. Both types can cause hyperkalemia. Beta-Adrenergic Blockers do not worsen renal function but, beyond blood pressure control, they do not protect the kidney (Hannedouche et al, 1994). Carvedilol is a Beta-Adrenergic Blocker with non-selective α_1 activity that displays some advantages: beneficial effects on lipid profile (Stafylas & Sarafidis, 2008), increase of insulin sensitivity, and the capacity to reduce albumin excretion (Bakris et al, 2004). Respecting renal hemodynamics, carvedilol preserves the renal blood flow and the glomerular filtation rate (GFR), whereas decreases the renal vascular resistance. Furthermore, has anti-oxidant activity. Contradictory results concerning the favorable effect of Beta-Adrenergic Blocker on cardiovascular morbidity and mortality of CKD patients have been reported in medical literature. Prospective RCT are needed to ascertain whether these anti-hypertensive drugs really do have a positive influence on the survival of renal patients or not. Aldosterone antagonists can be used in renal patients, but with great caution if the GFR is below 30 ml/min, the patient is taking an ACE inhibitor or an ARB, or has additional risk factors for hyperkaliemia. The association of aldosterone antagonists with AII antagonists is justified by the called aldosterone escape phenomenon. The hypothetical advantage of this add-on therapy is attributed to the anti-fibrotic and anti-hypertensive properties of aldosterone antagonists. Although there are some beneficial effects in terms of proteinuria , the addition of an aldosterone antagonist to an ACE inhibitor or to an ARB does not slow the progression of renal failure. Besides, the risk of hyperkalemia is markedly increased. Renin Inhibitors, a new class of antagonists of the RAS that blocks the conversion of angiotensinogen to angiotensin I, have recently started to be used worldwide. Aliskiren, the first compound of the class, shows an effective blood pressure control and reduces albuminuria successfully in type 2 diabetic patients, when given alone (Persson et al, 2009) or in combination with losartan (Parving et al, 2008). This renoprotection is independent of its blood pressure lowering effect. Further studies are needed to determine if aliskiren, alone or in association, is able to reduce hard renal and cardiovascular end-points in CKD patients. The utilization of α-adrenergic agents or the potent vasodilator minoxidil is only justified if blood pressure control was still not achieved with the previous described classes of anti-hypertensive drugs. They are extremely potent agents but present many adverse side effects. Furthermore, minoxidil must always be associated with a Beta-Adrenergic Blocker and a diuretic in order to control the reflex tachycardia and the fluid retention induced by the former (KDOQI, 2004).

4.2.4 What about the dual blockade of the RAS?

The rational for using two antagonists of the RAS is sustained by the existence of the AII escape phenomenon. After long-term ACE inhibition, it was demonstrated that AII synthesis via non-ACE pathways increases. Moreover, there are some limitations of ACE inhibitors in decreasing the local production of AII (Arici & Erdem, 2009). The ARB blocks the binding of AII to its receptors, reducing both its systemic and local effects (Arici & Erdem, 2009). There are advantages and drawbacks of combination therapy (Wolf & Ritz, 2005), but, in clinical terms, the aim of combination therapy is to block of the RAS more effectively (Arici & Erdem, 2009). Although several studies showed a greater decrease of albuminuria with the dual blockade (Mogensen et al, 2000; Campbell et al, 2003; Jennings et al, 2007), there are no RCT demonstrating a true slow down of CKD with combination therapy. In the ONTARGET study, the group of patients under ramipril plus telmisartan presented a higher renal impairment - doubling of serum creatinine or dialysis - and there were no differences in respect to cardiovascular outcomes (Yusuf et al, 2008). The ValHeFT and the VALIANT studies also showed more kidney dysfunction in the combination groups (Conn et al, 2001; Pfeffer et al, 2003), despite better cardiovascular results in the ValHeFT (Conn et al, 2001). In summary, concerning CKD progression, despite the theoretical advantages of combination therapy, presently there are no RCT demonstrating such benefit. Furthermore, the dual blockade is not harmless, and is associated with the risk of hyperkalemia and of greater renal impairment. Probably, studies with selected patients (with proteinuria > 1g/24h) or a different type of dual blockade with a renin inhibitor, will demonstrate a clear superiority of an association of two antagonists of the RAS. At the moment this association cannot be recommended.

5. Conclusion

Hypertension and CKD are both the chicken and the egg in this story. CKD resulting from hypertension and hypertension resulting from CKD are complex and multifactorial. A better understanding of the physiopathology mechanisms is imperative to improve our treatment strategies and reduce renal and cardiovascular adverse events. After decades of intense basic and clinical research in this area many questions remain unanswered: Is essential hypertension a cause of CKD in Caucasians? Which is the prevalent physiopathological mechanisms underlying CKD related hypertension in a particular patient? Which is the better anti-hypertensive therapy in our CKD patients and particularly in a specific patient?

6. References

Abbate, M. (1998). In progressive nephropathies, overload of tubular cells with filtered proteins translates glomerular permeability dysfunction into cellular signals of interstitial inflammation. J Am Soc Nephrol, Vol. 9, No.7, (July, 1998), pp. 1213-24

Acosta, J.H (1982). Hypertension in chronic renal disease. Kidney Int, Vol. 22, No.6, (December, 1982), pp. 702-712

Agodoa, L.Y. for the African American Study of Kidney Disease and Hypertension (AASK) Study Group (2001). Effect of ramipril vs amlodipine on renal outcomes in hypertensive nephrosclerosis: A randomized controlled trial. JAMA, Vol. 6, No. 285, Issue 21, (June, 2001), pp. 2719-2728

Appel, L.J. (2010). Intensive Blood-Pressure Control in Hypertensive Chronic Kidney Disease. N Engl J Med, Vol. 363, No.10, (September, 2010), pp. 918-929

Alvarez, V. (2002). Overload proteinuria is followed by salt sensitive hypertension caused by renal infiltration of immune cells. Am J Physiol Renal Physiol, Vol. 283, No. 5, (November, 2002), pp. F1132-F1141

Arici, M. (2009). Dual Blockade of the Renin-Angiotensin System for Cardio-renal Protection: An Update. Am J Kidney Dis, Vol. 53, No. 2, (February, 2009), pp. 332-345

August, P. (2000). Hypertension-induced organ damage in African Americans: transforming growth factor-beta (1) excess as a mechanism for increased prevalence. Curr Hypertens Rep, Vol. 2, No. 2, (April, 2000), pp. 184-191

Bakris, G.L. (1996). Calcium channel blockers versus other antihypertensive therapies on progression of NIDDM associated nephropathy. Kidney Int, Vol. 50, No. 5, (November, 1996), pp. 1641-1650

Bakris, G.L. (2004). Metabolic Effects of Carvedilol vs Metoprolol in Patients with Type 2 Diabetes Mellitus and Hypertension. A Randomized Controlled Trial. JAMA, Vol. 292, No. 18, (November, 2004), pp. 2227-2236.

Bakris, G.L. (2010). Renal outcomes with different fixed-dose combination therapies in patients with hypertension at high risk for cardiovascular events (ACCOMPLISH): a prespecified secondary analysis of a randomized controlled trial. Lancet, Vol. 375, No. 9721, (April, 2010), pp: 1173-1181

Balamuthusamy, S. (2008). Renin angiotensin system blockade and cardiovascular outcomes in patients with chronic kidney disease and proteinuria: a meta-analysis. Am Heart J, Vol. 155, No. 5, (May, 2008), pp. 791-805

Beretta-Piccoli, C. (1976). Hypertension associated with early stage kidney disease. Complementary roles of circulating renin, the body sodium/volume state and duration of hypertension. Am J Med, Vol. 61, (November, 1976), pp. 739-747

Bidani, A. K. (1994). Renal ablation acutely transforms "benign" hypertension to "malignant nephrosclerosis" in hypertensive rats. Hypertension, Vol. 24, No. 3, (September, 1994), pp. 309-316.

Bottinger, E.P. (2002). TGF-beta signaling in renal disease. J Am Soc Nephrol; Vol. 13, No. 10 (October, 2001), pp. 2600–2610

Brenner, B. M. (1985). Nephron adaptation to renal injury or ablation. American Journal of Physiology 249, F324-F337

Brenner, B.M. (2001). Effects of losartan on renal and cardiovascular outcomes in patients with type 2 diabetes and nephropathy. N Engl J Med, Vol. 345, No. 12, (September, 2001), pp. 861-869

Brown, D.M. (1996). Renal disease susceptibility and hypertension are under independent genetic control in the fawn-hooded rat. Nature Genet; Vol. 12, No. 1, (January, 1996), pp.44-51.

Caetano, E.P. (1999). The clinical diagnosis of hypertensive nephrosclerosis-how reliable is it? Nephrol Dial Transpl, Vol. 14, No. 2 (February, 1999), pp. 288-290.

Campbell, R. (2003). Effects of combined ACE inhibitor and angiotensin II antagonist treatment in human chronic nephropathies. Kidney Int, Vol. 63. No.3, (March, 2003), pp. 1094-103

Campese, V.M. (1991). Abnormal renal hemodynamics in black salt-sensitive patients with hypertension. Hypertension, Vol. 18, No. 6, (December, 1991), pp. 805–812

Carvalho,J.J. (1989). Blood pressure in four remote populations in the INTERSALT Study. Hypertension, Vol. 14, (September, 1989), pp. 238-246

Carlos, P. V. (2003). Local induction of angiotensin-converting enzyme in the kidney as a mechanism of progressive renal diseases. Kidney Int, Vol. 64, No. 86,suppl 86s, (October, 2003), pp. S57-S63

Casas, J.P. (2005). Effect of inhibitors of the renin-angiotensin system and other antihypertensive drugs on renal outcomes: systematic review and meta-analysis. Lancet, Vol. 366, No. 9502, (December, 2005), pp. 2026-2033

Casson, I.F. (1983). Failure of renal dopamine response to salt loading in chronic renal disease. Br Med J, Vol. 286, No. 6364, (February, 1983), 503-506

Chobanian, A.V. (2003). Joint Committee on Prevention, Definition, Evaluation and Treatment of High Blood Pressure. Hypertension, Vol. 42, No. 6, (December, 2003), pp. 1206-1256, ISSN 0194-911X

Chobanian, A. V. (1984). Recent advances in molecular pathology. The effects of hypertension on the arterial wall. Experimental and Molecular Pathology 41, 153-169.

Churchill, P.C. (1997). Genetic susceptibility to hypertension induced renal damage in the rat. Evidence based on kidney-specific genome transfer. J Clin Invest; Vol. 100, No. 6 (September, 1997), pp. 1373-1382

Cianciaruso, B. (1998). Salt intake and renal outcome in patients with progressive renal disease. Miner Electrolyte Metab Vol.24, No.4 (July-August, 1998), pp. 296-301

Cohn, J.N. (2001). A Randomized Trial of the Angiotensin-Receptor Blocker Valsartan in Chronic Heart Failure. N Engl J Med, Vol. 345, No. 23, (December, 2003), pp. 1667-1675

Coleman, T.G. (1969). Hypertension caused by salt loading in the dog. III. Onset transients of cardiac output and other circulatory variables. Circ Res, Vol. 25, (August, 1969), pp. 152-160, ISSN 0009-7330

Converse, R.L. (1992). Sympathetic overactivity in patients with chronic renal failure. N Engl J Med, Vol. 327, No. 27, (December, 1992), pp.1912-1918

Davies, D.L. (1973). Relationship between exchangeable sodium and the renin - angiotensin system and in hypertension with chronic renal failure. Lancet ,Vol. 301, No. 7805, (March, 1973), pp. 683-686

Duru, K. (1994). Frequency of a deletion polymorphism in the gene for angiotensin converting enzyme is increased in African Americans with hypertension. Am J Hypertens, Vol. 7, No. 8 (August, 1994), pp. 759-762

Dussaule, J.C. (2011). The role of cell palsticity in progression and reversal of renal fibrosis. Int. J. Path, Vol. 92, No. 3 (June, 2011), pp. 151-157

Eddy, A.A. (1995). Renal expression of genes that promote interstitial inflammation and fibrosis in rats with protein-overload proteinuria. Kidney Int, Vol. 47, No. 6, (June, 1995), pp. 1546-57

Ellis, A. W. M. (1942). The natural history of Bright's disease. Lancet i, 1-6, 34-38, 72-76.

Eng, E. (1994). Renal proliferative and phenotypic changes in rats with two kidney, one-clip Goldblatt hypertension. American Journal of Hypertension, Vol. 7, No.2, (February, 1994), pp. 177-185.

Estacio, R.O. (2000). Effect of blood pressure control on diabetic microvascular complications in patients with hypertension and type 2 diabetes. Diabetes Care, Vol. 23, Suppl.2, (April, 2000), pp. B54-64

Fine, .LG. (1998). Progressive renal disease: The chronic hypoxia hypothesis. Kidney Int, Vol. 53, No. , Suppl 65, (1998), pp. S74–S78.

Fisher, E. R. (1966). Ultrastructural studies in hypertension. I. Comparison of renal vascular and juxtaglomerular cell alterations in essential and renal hypertension in man. Laboratory Investigation 15, 1409-1433.

Fogo, A. (1997). Accuracy of the diagnosis of hypertensive nephrosclerosis in African Americans: a report from the African American Study of Kidney Disease (AASK) Trial. AASK Pilot Study Investigators. Kidney Int, Vol. 51, No. 1, (January, 1997), pp. 244-252.

Freedman, B.I. (1993). The familial risk of end-stage renal disease in African Americans. Am J Kidney Dis, Vol. 21, No.4 , (April, 1993), pp.387-393

Freedman, B.I. (1995). The link between hypertension and nephrosclerosis. Am J Kidney Dis, Vol. 25, No. 2, (February, 1995), pp.207–221

Freedman, B.I. (1998). Genetic initiation of hypertensive and diabetic nephropathy. Am J Hypertens, Vol. 11, No. 2, (February, 1998), pp. 251-257

Freedman, B.I. (2009). Plymorphisms in the non-muscle myosin heavy chain 9 gene (MYH9) are stongly associated with end-stage renal disease historically attributed to hypertension in African Americans. Kidney Int, Vol. 75, No. 7 (April, 2009), pp. 736-45

Fujihara, C.K. (1998). Mycophenolate mofetil attenuates renal injury in the rat remnant kidney. Kidney Int, Vol. 54, No. 5, (November, 1998), pp. 1510-9

Fujihara, C.K. (2000). Combined mycophenolate mofetil and losartan therapy arrests established injury in the remnant kidney. J Am Soc Nephrol, Vol. 11, No. 2, (February, 2000), pp. 283–290

Fung, M.M. (2009). Adenergic beta-1 receptor genetic variation predicts longitudinal rate of GFR decline in hypertensive nephrosclerosis. Nephrol Dial Transplant, Vol. 24, No. 12, (December, 2009), pp. 3677-86

Fung, M.M. (2011). Methylenetetrahydrofolate reductase (*MTHFR*) polymorphism A1298C (Glu429Ala) predicts decline in renal function over time in the African-American Study of Kidney Disease and Hypertension (AASK) Trial and Veterans Affairs Hypertension Cohort (VAHC). Nephrol Dial Transplant, (May, 2011) doi: 10.1093/ndt/gfr257

Goddard, J. (2004). Endothelin-A Receptor Antagonism Reduces Blood Pressure and Increases Renal Blood Flow in Hypertensive Patients with Chronic Renal Failure in CKD. Circulation Vol. 109, No. 9, (March, 2004), pp. 1186-1193

Goldblatt, H. (1964). Hypertension of renal origin. Historical and experimental background. American Journal of Surgery, Vol. 107, (January, 1964), pp. 21-25.

Gómez-Garre, D. (2001). Activation of NF-kB in tubular epithelial cells of rats with intense proteinuria. Role of angiotensin II and endothelin-1. Hypertens, Vol. 37, No.4, (April, 2001), pp. 1171-8

Guyton A.C. (1980). Salt Balance and long term pressure control. Annu Rev Med, Vol. 31, (February, 1980), pp. 15-27

Halimi, J.M. (2000). Renal effects of smoking: potential mechanisms and perspectives. Nephrol Dial Transplant, Vol.15, No. 7, (July, 2000), pp. 938-940

Hamlyn, J.M. (1996). Endogenous ouabain, sodium balance and blood pressure: a review and a hypothesis. J Hypertens, Vol. 13, No.2, (February, 1996), pp. 151-167

Hampton, J. A., (1989). Morphometric evaluation of the renal arterial system of Dahl salt-sensitive and salt-resistant rats on a high salt diet. II. Interlobular arteries and intralobular arterioles. Laboratory Investigation, Vol. 60, No. 6, (June, 1989), pp. 839-846.

Hannedouche, T. (1994). Randomised controlled trial of enalapril and beta blockers in non-diabetic chronic renal failure. Br Med J, Vol. 309, No. 6958, October, 1994), pp. 833-837.

Heeg, J.E. (1989). Efficacy and variability of the antiproteinuric effect of ACE inhibition by lisinopril. Kidney Int, Vol. 35, No.1, (January, 1989), pp. 272-279

Heerspink, H.J. (2010). Effects of a fixed combination of perindopril and indapamide in patients with type 2 diabetes and chronic kidney disease. Eur Heart J, Vol. 31, No. 23, (December, 2010), pp. 2888-2896

Helmchen, U. (1984). Intrarenal arteries in rats with early two-kidney, one clip hypertension. Hypertension,Vol. 6, 6PTt2 , (November-December, 1984), pp. III 87-92

Heptinstall, R. H. (1953). Malignant hypertension: a study of fifty-one cases. Journal of Pathology and Bacteriology, Vol. 65, No. 2, (April,1953), pp. 423-439

Higgins, D.F. (2007). Hypoxia promotes fibrogenesis in vivo via HIF-1 stimulation of epithelial-to-mesenchymal transition. J Clin Invest, Vol. 117, No. 12, (December, 2007), pp. 3810-3820

Hirsh, S. (2008). An update on proteinuric chronic kidney disease: The dual approach criteria. Cleveland Clinic Journal of Medicine, Vol. 75, No.10, (October, 2008), pp. 705-713

Hsu, C. (2005). Elevated blood pressure and risk for end-stage renal disease in subjects without baseline kidney disease. Arch Intern Med, Vol. 165, No. 8, (April, 2005), pp. 923–928

Hu, Q. (1998). Hydrogen peroxide induces intracellular calcium oscillations in human aortic endothelial cells. Circulation, Vol. 97, No. 3, (January, 1998), pp. 268-275, ISSN 0009-7322

Hung, A.M. (2010). CRP polymorphisms and progression of chronic kidney disease in African Americans. Clin J AM Soc Nephrol, Vol. 5, No. 1, (January, 2010), pp. 24-33

Jafar, T.H. (2001). Angiotensin-Converting Enzyme Inhibitors and Progression of Nondiabetic Renal Disease. A Meta-Analysis of Patient-Level Data. Ann Intern Med, Vol. 135, No.2, (July, 2001), pp. 73-87

Jafar, T.H. (2003). Progression of chronic kidney disease: the role of blood pressure control, proteinuria, and angiotensin-converting enzyme inhibition: a patient-level meta-analysis. Ann Intern Med, Vol. 139, No. 4, (August, 2003), pp. 244-252

Jennings, D.L. (2007). Combination therapy with an ACE inhibitor and an angiotensin receptor blocker for diabetic nephropathy: a meta-analysis. Diabetic Medicine, Vol. 24, No.5, (May, 2007), pp. 486-493

Johansen, K.L. (2007). Exercise in the End-Stage Renal disease Population. J Am Soc Nephrol, Vol. 18, No.6, (June, 2007), pp. 1845-1854

Joint Specialty Committee on Renal Medicine of the Royal College of Physicians and the Renal Association, and the Royal College of General Practitioners. Chronic Kidney Disease in Adults: UK Guidelines for Identification, Management and Referral. London. Royal College of Physicians. 2006, ISBN 1 86016 276 2, London, United Kingdom

Kaplan, N.M. (2006a) Hypertension in the Population at Large. In Clinical Hypertension, N.M. Kaplan & J.T. Flynn (Eds.), 1-24, Lippincott Williams and Wilkins, ISBN 0-7817-6198-0, Philadelphia, USA

Kaplan, N.M. (2006b). Treatment of Hypertension: Drug Therapy, In: Clinical Hypertension. N.M. Kaplan & J.T. Flynn (Eds.), 217-230, Lippincott Williams and Wilkins, ISBN 0-7817-6198-0, Philadelphia, USA

Kearney, P. M. (2004). Worldwide prevalence of hypertension: a systematic review. J. Hypertens, Vol. 22, No. 1, (January, 2004), pp.11–19

Kearney, P. M. (2005). Global burden of hypertension: analysis of worldwide data. Lancet, Vol. 365, No. 9455, (January, 2005), pp. 217–223

Kincaid-Smith, P. S. (1982). Renal hypertension. In Hypertension - Mechanisms and Management (ed. P. S. Kincaid-Smith and J. A. Whitworth), pp. 94-101. New York: ADIS Health Science Press, 1982

Kincaid-Smith, P. (1999). Clinical diagnosis of hypertensive nephrosclerosis. Nephrol Dial Transplant, Vol. 14, No. 9, (September, 1999), pp. 2255–2256

Klag, M. J. (1996). Blood pressure and end-stage renal disease in men. N Engl J Med, Vol. 334, No. 1, (January, 1996), pp. 13–18

Klag, M.J. (1997). End-stage Renal Disease in African-American and White Men: 16-Year MRFIT Findings, JAMA, Vol. 277, No. 16 (April, 1997), pp. 1293-1298

Klahr, S. (1988). The progression of renal disease. N Engl J Med, Vol. 318, No. 25, (June, 1988), pp. 1657-1666.

Klahr, S. (1994). The effects of dietary protein restriction and blood-pressure control on the progression of chronic kidney disease. N Engl J Med, Vol. 330, No. 13, (March, 1994), pp. 877-884

Klemperer, P. (1931). Malignant nephrosclerosis (Fahr). Archives of Pathology 11, 60-117

KDOQI (2004). Clinical Practice Guidelines on Hypertension and Antihypertensive Agents in Chronic Kidney Disease. Am J Kidney Dis, Vol. 43, Suppl. 1, (May, 2004), pp. S65-S230

Khawaja, Z. (2011). Role of the Kidneys in Resistant Hypertension. Int J Hypertens, Vol. 2011, Article ID 143471, 8 pages, 2011. doi:10.4061/2011/143471

Komiyama, Y. (2005). A novel endogenous digitalis, telecinobufagin, exhibits elevated plasma levels in patients with terminal renal failure. Clin Biochem, Vol. 38, No.1, (January, 2005), pp. 36-45

Largo, R. (1999). Angiotensin-converting enzyme is upregulated in the proximal tubules of rats with intense proteinuria. Hypertens, Vol. 33, No. 3, (Febryuary 1999), pp. 732–739.

Lee, R. M. K. W. (1987). Structural alterations of blood vessels in hypertensive rats. Canadian Journal of Physiology and Pharmacology 65, 1528-1538

Leh, S. (2011). Afferent arteriolopathy and glomerular collapse but not segmental sclerosis induce tubular atrophy in old spontaneously hypertensive rats. Virchows Arch, Vol. 459, No. 1, (July, 2011), pp. 99-108

Leone, A. (1972). Accumulation of an endogenous inhibitor of nitric oxide synthesis in chronic renal failure. Lancet, Vol. 340, No. 8793, (March, 1992), pp. 572-575

Levin, A. (2008). Guidelines for the management of chronic kidney disease. CMAJ, Vol. 179, No.11, (November, 2008), pp.1154-1162

Lewis, E.J. (1993). The effect of angiotensin-converting-enzyme inhibitor on diabetic nephropathy. N Engl J Med 1993, Vol. 329, No. 20, (November, 1993), pp. 1456-1462

Lewis, E.J. (2001). Renoprotective effect of angiotensin receptor antagonist irbersartan in patients with nephropathy due to type 2 diabetes. N Engl J Med, Vol. 345, No. 12, (September, 2001), pp. 851-860

Luft, F. C. (1995). Hypertension-induced renal injury: is mechanically mediated interstitial inflammation involved? Nephrol Dial Transplant, Vol. 10, No. 1, (January, 1995), pp. 9-11

Mailloux, L.U. (2001). Hypertension in chronic renal failure and ESRD: Prevalence, pathophysiology, and outcomes. Semin Nephrol, Vol. 21, No.2, (March, 2001), pp. 146-156

Makki, D.D.(1995). Long-term effects of antihypertensive agents on proteinuria and renal function. Arch Intern Med, Vol. 155, No.10, (May, 1995), pp. 1073-1080

Mann, J.F. (2001). Renal insufficiency as a predictor of cardiovascular outcomes and the impact of ramipril: The HOPE randomized trial. Ann Intern Med, Vol. 134, No.8, (April, 2001), pp. 629 -636

Marcantoni, C. (2002). Hypertensive nephrosclerosis in African Americans versus Caucasians. Kidney Int, Vol. 62, No. 1, (July, 2002), pp. 172-180

Mayer, G. (1993). Effects of angiotensin II receptor blockade on remnant glomerular permselectivity. Kidney Int, Vol. 43, No. 2, (February, 1993), pp. 346-353

Mazzali, M. (2001). Elevated uric acid increases blood pressure in the rat by a novel crystal independent mechanism. Hypertens, Vol. 38, No. 5, (November, 2001), pp.1101–1106

Meguid El Nahas, A. (2005). Chronic kidney disease: the global challenge. Lancet, Vol. 365, No. 9456 , (January, 2005), pp. 331–340

Mogensen, C.E. (1976). Progression of nephropathy in long-term diabetics with proteinuria and effect of initial anti-hypertensive treatment. Scand J Clin Lab Invest, Vol. 36, No. 4, (July, 1976), pp. 383–388

Mogensen, C.E. (2000). Randomised controlled trial of dual blockade of renin-angiotensin system in patients with hypertension, microalbuminuria, and non-insulin dependent diabetes: the candesartan and lisinopril microalbuminuria (CALM) study. Br Med J, Vol. 321, No. 7274, (December, 2000), pp. 1440-1444

Müller, D.N. (2000). NF-κB inhibition ameliorates angiotensin II–induced inflammatory damage in rats. Hypertens, Vol. 35, No. 1 Pt 2, (January, 2000), pp. 193–201

Müller, D.N. (2001). Aspirin inhibits NF-κB and protects from angiotensin II-induced organ damage. FASEB J, Vol. 15, No. 10, (August, 2001), pp. 1822–1824

Mulvany, M. J. (1990). Structure and function of small arteries. Physiological Reviews, Vol. 70, No. 4, (October, 1990), pp. 921-961

Nathan, S. (2005). Effects on Cardio-Renal Risk in Hypertensive Patients. Hypertension, Vol. 46, No. 4, (October, 2005), pp. 637-642, ISSN 0194-911X

Navar, L.G. (1996). Interactions between arterial pressure and sodium excretion. Curr Opin Nephrol Hypertens Vol. 5, (1996), pp. 64-71

Neves, P.L. (2007). Anaemia correction in predialysis elderly patients: influence of the antihypertensive therapy on darbepoietin dose. Int Urol Nephrol, Vol.39, No. 2, (June, 2007), pp. 685-689

Nordborg, C. (1983). Morpho-metric study of mesenteric and renal arteries in spontaneously hypertensive rats. Journal of Hypertension, Vol. 1, No. 4, (December, 1983), pp. 333-338

Ong, A. C. M. (1994). Loss of glomerular function and tubulointerstitial fibrosis: cause or effect? Kidney Int, Vol. 45, No. 2, (February, 1994), pp. 345-351.

Ong, K. L (2007). Prevalence, awareness and treatment of hypertension among United States adults 1999–2004. Hypertension, Vol. 49, No. 1, (January, 2007), pp. 69–75

Orth, S.R. (2003). Cigarette smoking: an important renal risk factor - far beyond carcinogenesis. Tobacco Induced Diseases, Vol. 1, No.2, (June, 2003), pp. 137-155

Owens, G. K. (1982). Alterations in vascular smooth muscle mass in the spontaneously hypertensive rat. Role of cellular hyper-trophy, hyperploidy, and hyperplasia. Circulation Research, Vol. 51, No. 3 , (September, 1982), pp.9280-289.

Page, I. Renal Hypertension. Chicago, IL: Year Book, 1968.

Parving, H.H. (2008). Aliskiren Combined with Losartan in Type 2 Diabetes and Nephropathy. N Engl J Med, Vol. 358, No. 23, (June, 2008), pp. 2433-2446

Perneger, T.V. (1995). Diagnosis of hypertensive end stage renal disease: Effect of patients'race. Am J Epidemiol., Vol. 141, No. 1, (January, 1995), pp.10-15

Perry, H. M. (1995). Early predictors of 15-year end-stage renal disease in hypertensive patients. Hypertension, Vol. 25, No. 4 Pt 1, (April, 1995), pp. 587–594

Persson, F. (2009). Renal Effects of Aliskiren Compared With and in Combination With Irbersartan in Patients With Type 2 Diabetes, Hypertension, and Albuminuria. Diabetes Care, Vol. 32, No.10, (October, 2009), pp. 1873-1879

Pestana, M. (2001). Renal Dopaminergic mechanisms in renal parenchymal diseases and hypertension. Nephrol Dial Transplant 2001, Vol. 16, Suppl. 1, (May, 2001), pp. 53-59

Pfeffer, M.A. (2003). Valsartan, Captopril, or Both in Myocardial Infarction Complicated by Heart Failure, Left Ventricular Dysfunction, or Both. N Engl J Med, Vol. 349, No. 20, (November, 2003), pp.1893-1906

Pohl, M.A. (2005). Independent and Additive Impact of Blood Pressure Control and Angiotensin II Receptor Blockade on Renal Outcomes in the Irbesartan Diabetic Nephropathy Trial: Clinical Implications and Limitations. J Am Soc Nephrol, Vol. 16, No. 10, (October, 2005), pp. 3027-3037

Praga, M. (2006). Weight loss and proteinuria. In: Obesity and the Kidney, G. Wolf (Ed.), pp. 221-229, ISBN 10:3-8055-1164-5

Rettig, R. (1990). Hypertension in rats induced by renal grafts from reno-vascular hypertensive donors. Hypertension 15, 429-435.

Ridao, N. (2001). Prevalence of Hypertension in Renal Disease. Nephrol Dial Transplant, Vol. 16, Suppl. 1 (May, 2001), pp. 70-73

Romero, F. (1999). Mycophenolate mofetil prevents the progressive renal failure induced by 5/6 renal ablation in rats. Kidney Int, Vol. 55, No. 3, (March, 1999), pp. 945–955.

Ross, R. (1993). The pathogenesis of atherosclerosis: a perspective for the 1990s. Nature, Vol. 362, No. 6423, (April, 1993), pp. 801-809

Rosenberg, M.E. (1994). The paradox of the renin-angiotensin system in chronic renal disease. Kidney Int. Vol. 45, No. 2, (February, 1994), pp. 403-410

Rostand, S. G. (1982). Racial differences in the incidence of treatment for end-stage renal disease. N Engl J Med, Vol. 306, No.21 , (May, 1982), pp. 1276-1279.

Ruggenenti, P. (2000). The role of protein traffic in the progression of renal diseases. Annu Rev Med 2000, Vol. 51, (February, 2000), pp. 315–327

Ruggenenti, P. (2005). Blood-pressure control for renoprotection in patients with non-diabetic chronic renal disease (REIN-2): multicentre, randomised controlled trial. Lancet Vol. 365, No. 9463, (March, 2005), pp. 939-946

Rump, L.C. (2000). Sympathetic overactivity in renal disease: a window to understand progression and cardiovascular complications of uremia? Nephrol Dial Transplant 2000; Vol. 15, No. 11, (November, 2000), pp. 1735-1738

Sacks, F.M. (2001). Effects on blood pressure of reduced dietary sodium and the Dietary Approaches to Stop Hypertension (DASH) diet. DASH-Sodium Collaborative Research Group. N Engl J Med, Vol. 344, No.1, (January, 2001), pp. 3-10

Schoenborn, C. (2009). Health characteristics of adults aged 55 years and over: United States, 2004–2007. Natl Health Stat Report, Vol. 8, No. 16, (July, 2008), pp. 1-31

Shulman, N.B. (1989). Prognostic value of serum creatinine and effect of treatment of hypertension on renal function . Results from the hypertension detection and follow-up program. Hypertension, Vol 13, Suppl I, (May 1989), pp. I80-I93

Sica, D.A. (2003). Combination Angiotensin Converting Enzyme Inhibitor and Angiotensin Receptor Blocker Therapy: It's Role in Clinical Practice. J Clin Hypertens, Vol. 4, No. 6, (November-December, 2003), pp. 414-420

Sica, D. (2005). Pathological Basis and Treatment Considerations in Chronic Kidney Disease - Related Hypertension. Semin Nephrol Vol. 25, No. 4, (July, 2005), pp. 246-251

Sies, H. (1997). Oxidative Stress: oxidants and anti-oxidants. Exp Physiol, Vol.82, No.2, (March, 1997), pp. 291-295

Sleight, P. (2009). Prognostic value of blood pressure in patients with high vascular risk in the Ongoing Telmisartan Alone and in combination with Ramipril Global Endpoint Trial study. J Hypertens, Vol. 27, (July, 2009), pp. 1360-1369

Solomon, S.D. (2006). Renal Function and Effectiveness of Angiotensin-Converting Enzyme Inhibitor Therapy in Patients With Chronic Stable Coronary Disease in the Prevention of Events with ACE inhibition (PEACE) Trial. Circulation, Vol 114, No. 1, (July, 2006), pp. 26-31 ISSN 0009; 7322

Sommers, S. C. (1958). Histologic studies of kidney biopsy specimens from patients with hypertension. American Journal of Pathology, Vol 34, No. 4, (July-August, 1958), pp. 685-715

Stafylas, P.C. (2008). Carvedilol in hypertension treatment. Vasc Health Risk Manag, Vol. 4, No. 1, (March, 2008), pp. 23–30.

Suter, P.M. (2008). The effect of exercise, alcohol or both combined on health and physical performance. Alcohol metabolism during exercise. Int J Obesity. Vol. 32, (December, 2008), pp. S48-S52

Suthanthiran, M. (1998). Transforming growth factor-beta 1 hyperexpression in African American end-stage renal disease patients. Kidney Int, Vol. 53, No. 3, (March 1998), pp. 639-644

Takahashi, H. (2011). The central mechanism underlying hypertension: a review of sodium ions, epithelial sodium channels, the renin-angiotensin-aldosterone system, oxidative stress and endogenous digitalis in the brain. *Hypertension Research* doi:10.1038/hr.2011.105

Takase, O. (2003). Gene transfer of truncated IkBa prevents tubulointerstitial injury. Kidney Int, Vol. 63, No.2 , (February, 2003), pp. 501-513

Tian, N. (2008). NAPDH oxidase contributes to renal damage and dysfunction in Dahl salt-sensitive hypertension. Am J Physiol Regul Integr Comp Physiol, Vol. 295, No. 6, (October, 2008), pp.R1858-R1865

Tomson, C. R. V. (1991). Does treated essential hypertension result in renal impairment? A cohort study. Journal of Human Hypertension, Vol. 5, No. 3, (June, 1991), pp. 189-192

Tracy, R.E. (1991). Blood pressure and nephrosclerosis in black and white men and women aged 25 to 54. Modern Pathol, Vol. 4, No.5 , (September, 1991), pp.602–609

Upadhyay, A. (2011). Systematic Review: Blood Pressure Target in Chronic Kidney Disease and Proteinuria as an Effect Modifier. Ann Intern Med, Vol. 155, No. 3, (August, 2011), pp. 207-208

US Renal data System, USRDS 2003 Annual report: Atlas of Chronic Kidney Disease and End-stage Renal Disease in the United States, NIH, NIDDKD, 2003.

US Renal data System, USRDS 2010 Annual report: Atlas of Chronic Kidney Disease and End-stage Renal Disease in the United States, NIH, NIDDKD, 2010

Valenzuela, R. (1980). Hyaline arteriolar nephrosclerosis. Immunofluorescence findings in the vascular lesions. Laboratory Investigation, Vol. 43, No. 6, (December, 1980), pp. 530-534

Van Bemmel, T. (2006). Prospective study of the effect of blood pressure on renal function in old age: the Leiden 85-Plus Study. J Am Soc Nephrol, Vol. 17, No. 9, (September, 2006), pp. 2561-2566

Vaziri, N.D. (1997). Altered nitric oxide metabolism and increased oxygen free radical activity in lead-induced hypertension: effect of lazaroid therapy. Kidney Int, Vol 52, No. 4, (October, 1997), pp. 1042-1046

Vaziri, N.D (2002). Enhanced nitric oxide inativation and protein nitration by reactive oxygen species in renal insufficiency. Hypertension, Vol. 39, No.1, (January, 2002), pp. 135-141

Vial, J. H. (1989). Histometric assessment of renal arterioles during DOCA and post-DOCA hypertension and hydralazine treatment in rats. Journal of Hypertension, Vol. 7, No. 3, (March, 1989), pp. 203-209.

Weisstuch, J. M. (1992). Does essential hypertension cause end-stage renal disease? Kidney Int, Vol. 41, Suppl. 36, (May, 1992), pp. S33-S37.

Wenzel, U. O. (2002). Repetitive application of anti Thy-1 antibody aggravates damage in the nonclipped but not in the clipped kidney of rats with Goldblatt hypertension. Kidney Int, Vol. 61, No. 6, (June, 2002), pp. 2119-2131.

Wolf, G. (2005). Combination therapy with ACE inhibitors and angiotensin II receptor blockers to halt the progression of chronic renal disease: Pathophysiology and indications. Kidney Int, Vol. 67, No. 3, (March, 2005), pp. 799-812

Wong, C. (2008). Genetic polymorphisms of the RAS-cytokine pathway and chronic kidney disease. Pediatr Nephrol , Vol 23, No.7, (July, 2008), pp. 1037-1051.

Wright, J.T. Jr. (2002). Effect of blood pressure lowering and antihypertensive drug class on progression of hypertensive kidney disease: results from the AASK trial. JAMA, 2002, Vol. 288, (November, 2002), pp. 2421-2431

Yang, J.W. (). Gene polymorphisms of vascular endothelial growth factor-1154 G>A is associated with hypertensive nephropathy in a hispanic population. Mol Biol Rep, Vol. 38, No. 4, (April, 2011), pp. 2417-25

Yu, H. (2002). Association of the tissue kallikrein gene promoter with ESRD and hypertension. Kidney Int, Vol. 61, No.3, (March, 2002), pp.1030-1039

Yusuf, S. (2008). Telmisartan, Ramipril, or Both in Patients at High Risk for Vascular Events. The ONTARGET Investigators. N Engl J Med, Vol. 358, No. 15, (April, 2008), pp. 1547-1559

Zarif, L. (2000). Inaccuracy of clinical pheno-typing parameters for hypertensive nephrosclerosis. Nephrol Dial Transplant, Vol. 15, No. 11, (November, 2000), pp. 1801-1807

Zoja, C. (1998). Protein overload stimulated RANTES production by proximal tubular cells depending on NF-kB activation. Kidney Int, Vol. 53, No. 6, (June, 1998), pp. 1608-1605

Zucchelli, P. (1995). Can we accurately diagnose nephrosclerosis? Nephrol Dial Transplant, Vol. 10, Suppl 6, (1995), pp. 2–5.

Zuchelli, P. (1998). Progression of renal failure and hypertensive nephrosclerosis. Kidney Int, Vol. 54, Suppl 68, (December, 1998), pp. S55 -S59

4

Potassium-Sparing Diuretics in Hypertension

Cristiana Catena, GianLuca Colussi and Leonardo A. Sechi
Clinica Medica, Department of Experimental and Clinical Medicine, University of Udine, Italy

1. Introduction

Abbreviations and acronyms in this chapter.

ENaC: amiloride-sensitive epithelial sodium channel; ROMK: renal outer medullary K channel; BK K^+: flow-sensitive maxi K channel; AQP-2: apical aquaporin; AQP-3 and 4: basolateral aquaporin; 11β-HSD2: 11β-hydroxysteroid dehydrogenase; NAD: nicotinamide adenine dinucleotide; ROS: reactive oxygen species; CYP11B2: aldosterone synthase; GPR30: G protein coupled receptor; PI3K: phosphatidylinositol 3-kinase; ERK: extracellular signal-regulated kinase; NYHA: New York Heart Association; HFPSF: heart failure and preserved systolic function (HFPSF); ACE: angiotensin-converting enzyme; CCB: calcium-channel blockers.

Many clinical studies have reported that cardiovascular morbidity and mortality have a continuous relationship with both systolic and diastolic blood pressures. Although some of these studies have reported that this relationship is steeper for stroke, in some European countries the attributable risk, that is the excess of events due to increased blood pressure, appears to be greater for coronary artery disease (Prospective Studies Collaboration, 2002). Current evidence indicates that both systolic and diastolic blood pressure levels have a continuous and independent relationship with a variety of additional organ complications, including congestive heart failure, renal failure, and peripheral artery disease. The wide prevalence of hypertension in the general population (Wolf-Maier et al. 2003) explains why hypertension has been identified as the first cause of death worldwide by the World Health Organization. This is also why today hypertension is considered as the most important correctable risk factor for cardiovascular diseases.

Recent guidelines have put strong emphasis on the relevance of hypertension-related subclinical organ damage and have prescribed that signs of organ involvement should be sought with great care. In fact, a large body of evidence indicates that hypertensive subclinical organ damage, including left ventricular hypertrophy, microalbuminuria, and thickening of inner vascular layers, is critical in determining the cardiovascular risk of individuals with high blood pressure (The Task Force for the Management of Arterial Hypertension of the European Society of Hypertension and of the European Society of Cardiology, 2007). In patients with high blood pressure, left ventricular hypertrophy has been shown repeatedly to be associated with an increased incidence of cardiovascular events, and similar evidence has been obtained for carotid intima-media thickening and microalbuminuria. Also and most important, prospective studies have demonstrated that reduction in left ventricular mass, intima-media thickness, and urinary protein excretion induced by antihypertensive treatment are associated with reduced incidence of cardiovascular events. This indicates that assessment of subclinical organ damage is critical not only for quantification of the cardiovascular risk, but also to monitor the beneficial effects of treatment. Large clinical trials that have evaluated the effects of blockade of the renin-angiotensin system with angiotensin-converting enzyme inhibitors or angiotensin receptor blockers have demonstrated a specific ability of these agents in preventing progression and inducing regression of hypertension-related subclinical organ damage. It must be noticed, however, that a significant percentage of hypertensive patients with left ventricular hypertrophy fail to achieve full regression of left ventricular mass when treated with renin-angiotensin system blockers, a fact that might be ascribed to plasma aldosterone escape from the inhibitory effect of these drugs. This hypothesis received the support of studies in which it was demonstrated that with use of renin-angiotensin system blockers left ventricular mass does not decrease in hypertensive patients with aldosterone escape as opposed to a decline in left ventricular mass that is observed in patients without aldosterone escape.

Several randomized controlled trials have tested the benefits of blood pressure lowering treatment providing undisputable evidence. Also, several meta-analyses that have collected an impressive number of patients have confirmed the evidence of benefits of treatment in event-based trials comparing active treatment with placebo, different active treatments, and more or less intense blood pressure lowering strategies. Findings of all these studies indicate that: a) use of antihypertensive drugs causes significant reductions of cardiovascular morbidity and mortality; b) reduction of cardiovascular risk is comparable in hypertensive patients of different ethnicity; c) the benefit of antihypertensive treatment is evident even in the elderly patients with isolated systolic hypertension; d) relative reduction of risk is greater for stroke (approximately 35%) than for coronary artery disease (approximately 20%). Overall, studies comparing different types of antihypertensive drugs show that differences in the incidence of cardiovascular morbidity and mortality are not relevant in the presence of comparable blood pressure reduction, thus supporting the conclusion that benefits of treatment are largely dependent on blood pressure reduction *per se*.

Diuretics decrease the total body pool of sodium-chloride and are included among the five major classes of antihypertensive agents that are suitable for the initiation and maintenance of antihypertensive treatment alone or in combination. This is due to the evidence of effective blood pressure lowering and effective prevention of cardiovascular events that has been obtained with thiazide diuretics. Current guidelines indicate congestive heart failure, isolated systolic hypertension, hypertension in blacks, and end-stage renal disease (this for loop diuretics) as conditions favoring use of diuretics versus other antihypertensive drugs. However, side effect of these drugs including decrease in plasma potassium, and increase in plasma glucose, cholesterol, triglyceride, and uric acid are important limiting factors.

Other classes of diuretics that are used in hypertension as monotherapy, but more frequently as combinations, are the so-called potassium-sparing diuretics. These include a group of drugs that act with different mechanisms at the distal tubular site of the nephron where the mineralocorticoid receptors are expressed and mediate the tubular effects of aldosterone and other mineralocorticoid hormones. The aldosterone-sensitive tubular site of the distal tubule handles only a small amount of sodium chloride and this is why the natriuretic effect of agents acting at this site is relatively modest. However, this tubular site contributes greatly to regulation of body potassium content and acid-base equilibrium by modulation of exchange of sodium with either potassium or hydrogen ions.

Aldosterone is a steroid hormone that is secreted by the zona glomerulosa of the adrenal cortex and is involved in regulation of blood pressure exerting its main effects on the distal tubular site of the nephron where it increases water and sodium chloride reabsorption thereby leading to expansion of the extracellular fluid volume. Recent views indicate that, in addition to its renal effects and regulatory role on body water and electrolyte balance, aldosterone acts on a variety of cell types affecting cellular mechanisms that mediate important tissue responses, including hypertrophy and fibrosis. Recent evidence obtained from experimental animal studies indicates that chronic exposure to inappropriately high aldosterone levels or activation of the mineralocorticoid receptors can induce tissue damage in specific organ sites with mechanisms that are independent of blood pressure elevation. These animal studies have demonstrated that tissue damage can be prevented by removal of adrenal glands or administration of aldosterone antagonists.

Spironolactone and eplerenone (Figure 1) are mineralocorticoid receptor antagonists commonly employed to reduce blood pressure, left ventricular hypertrophy, and urinary albumin excretion in patients with essential hypertension or primary aldosteronism. The latter effects occur beyond what is expected from the mere reduction of blood pressure, suggesting that activation of the mineralocorticoid receptor plays a central role in the development of cardiac and renal abnormalities in hypertensive patients. In agreement with

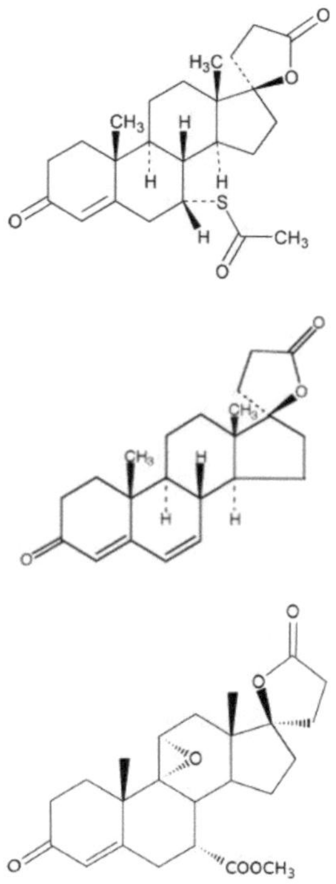

Spironolactone

Canrenone

Eplerenone

Fig. 1. Structure of the mineralocorticoid receptor antagonists currently available for clinical use

these findings, currently available evidence strongly supports the notion that aldosterone receptor antagonists are of considerable therapeutic value in patients with systolic heart failure with a cardioprotective effect that is already appreciable in the early functional stages. Also, recent evidence suggests that the benefits of aldosterone antagonists in the context of cardiac failure are not restricted to patients with impaired systolic function but can be extrapolated also to patients with diastolic dysfunction. Finally, some studies support the view that mineralocorticoid receptor blockade may exert an antialbuminuric effect in patients with proteinuria, an effect that occurs independent of blood pressure reduction.

The use of classic mineralocorticoid receptor antagonists, however, has been limited by the high incidence of breast engorgement and gynecomastia and the risk of severe hyperkalemia. To overcome these tolerance problems, new aldosterone blockers have been developed (Garthwaite & McMahon 2004) using two different strategies that include search for non-steroidal antagonists and inhibition of aldosterone synthesis. Inhibition of aldosterone synthesis could have an additional benefit due to blockade of the mineralocorticoid receptor-independent pathways that might account for some of the untoward effects of aldosterone. The new aldosterone blockers are currently having extensive preclinical evaluation, and one of them has passed phase-II trials showing promising results in patients with essential hypertension and primary aldosteronism.

2. Regulation of potassium excretion at the distal tubular site

More than 98% of total body potassium is located inside the cells and homeostatic control of extracellular potassium by the intracellular pool is critical in the regulation of plasma potassium concentration. Plasma potassium levels are maintained stable between 3.5 and 5.0 mEq/l despite remarkable variability in potassium intake with meals. This balance is due to mechanisms that operate principally at the renal level and regulate potassium excretion. In normal conditions, daily intake of potassium is entirely eliminated by the body, 90% by the kidney and 10% by the intestine. Therefore, changes in body potassium content are physiologically regulated by the kidney that compensates with increased reabsorption in conditions of hypokalemia, and increased secretion in conditions of hyperkalemia. Potassium transport occurs along the entire nephron, but the major role in potassium secretion is played at the distal site by the connecting tubule and cortical collecting duct. In these sites, principal cells are responsible for regulation of sodium reabsorption and via the amiloride-sensitive epithelial sodium channel (ENaC) (Figure 2) with the associated potassium and hydrogen ion excretion. Sodium entry via ENaC generates an excess of negative charges in the tubular lumen that causes intracellular potassium to leave the cell through the renal outer medullary K channel (ROMK) and the flow-sensitive maxi-K potassium channel (BK K^+) (Figure 2). In addition to distal sodium reabsorption through the ENaC, potassium secretion is therefore dependent on distal tubular flow. Aldosterone has direct influence on potassium secretion, activating sodium transport through activation of the ENaC and increasing the driving force for potassium secretion into the tubular lumen (Figure 3).

3. Mechanisms of aldosterone-induced tissue damage

A growing body of evidence suggests that exposure to inappropriate aldosterone levels for salt status or activation of the mineralocorticoid receptor can produce massive myocardial, vascular, and renal tissue injury with mechanisms that are independent of blood pressure (Marney & Brown, 2007). Landmark experiments demonstrated that chronic aldosterone infusion causes myocardial fibrosis in rats that are maintained on a high-salt diet. Later on, it was demonstrated that aldosterone-induced myocardial fibrosis is preceded by inflammatory changes of perivascular tissue, and that both inflammation and fibrosis can be prevented by administration of mineralocorticoid receptor antagonists or adrenalectomy. Similar evidence was obtained in the kidney of uninephrectomized and stroke-prone spontaneously hypertensive rats in which aldosterone produced intrarenal vascular damage, glomerular injury, and tubulointerstitial fibrosis. Elevated aldosterone also caused aortic fibrosis and hypertrophy in different rat models of hypertension, and administration of eplerenone to hypertensive rats corrected vascular remodeling and fibrosis, suggesting a mineralocorticoid receptor-mediated mechanism.

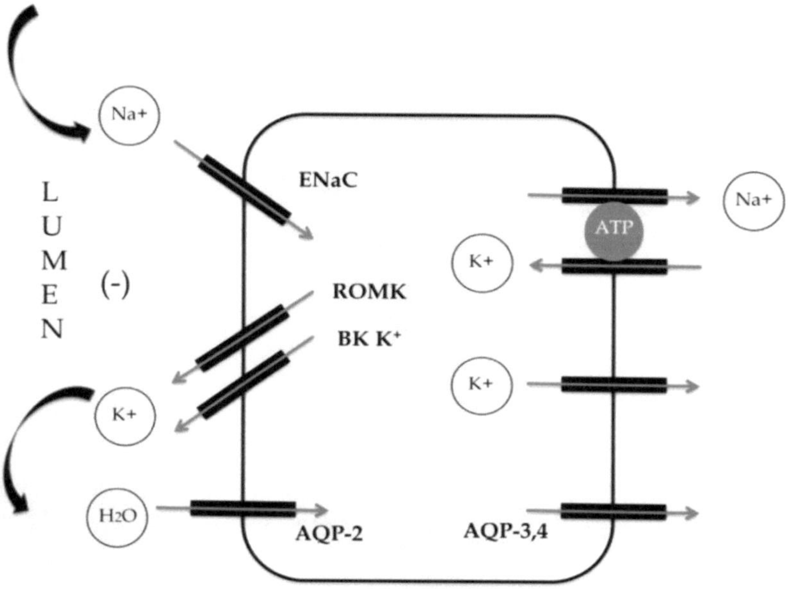

Fig. 2. Sodium, potassium, and water transport in principal cells of connecting tubule and cortical collecting duct. ENaC: amiloride-sensitive epithelial sodium channel; ROMK: renal outer medullary K channel; BK K^+: flow-sensitive maxi K channel; AQP-2: apical aquaporin; AQP-3 and 4: basolateral aquaporin.

All these studies consistently indicate that aldosterone causes tissue damage only in the context of inappropriate salt status. It was suggested that untoward effects of high-salt intake are largely dependent on activation of mineralocorticoid receptors and that this activation might reflect increased oxidative stress. Mineralocorticoid receptors are found in epithelial and nonepithelial tissues with high affinity for aldosterone and glucocorticoid hormones, such as cortisol and corticosterone. Under physiological conditions, the majority of mineralocorticoid receptors in nonepithelial tissues are occupied by greater concentrations of cortisol, whereas in epithelial tissues, binding of cortisol to receptors is prevented by 11β-hydroxysteroid dehydrogenase (11β-HSD2), the enzyme that converts cortisol to the receptor-inactive cortisone. In addition to the conversion of cortisol to cortisone, activity of 11β-HSD2 generates NADH from NAD and produces changes in the intracellular redox potential that might, in turn, inactivate the glucocorticoid–receptor complex. 11β-HSD2 is not present in nonepithelial tissues including the heart, but in such tissues, changes of the intracellular redox potential can result from generation of reactive oxygen species (ROS) and thereby affect the activity of the mineralocorticoid receptor.

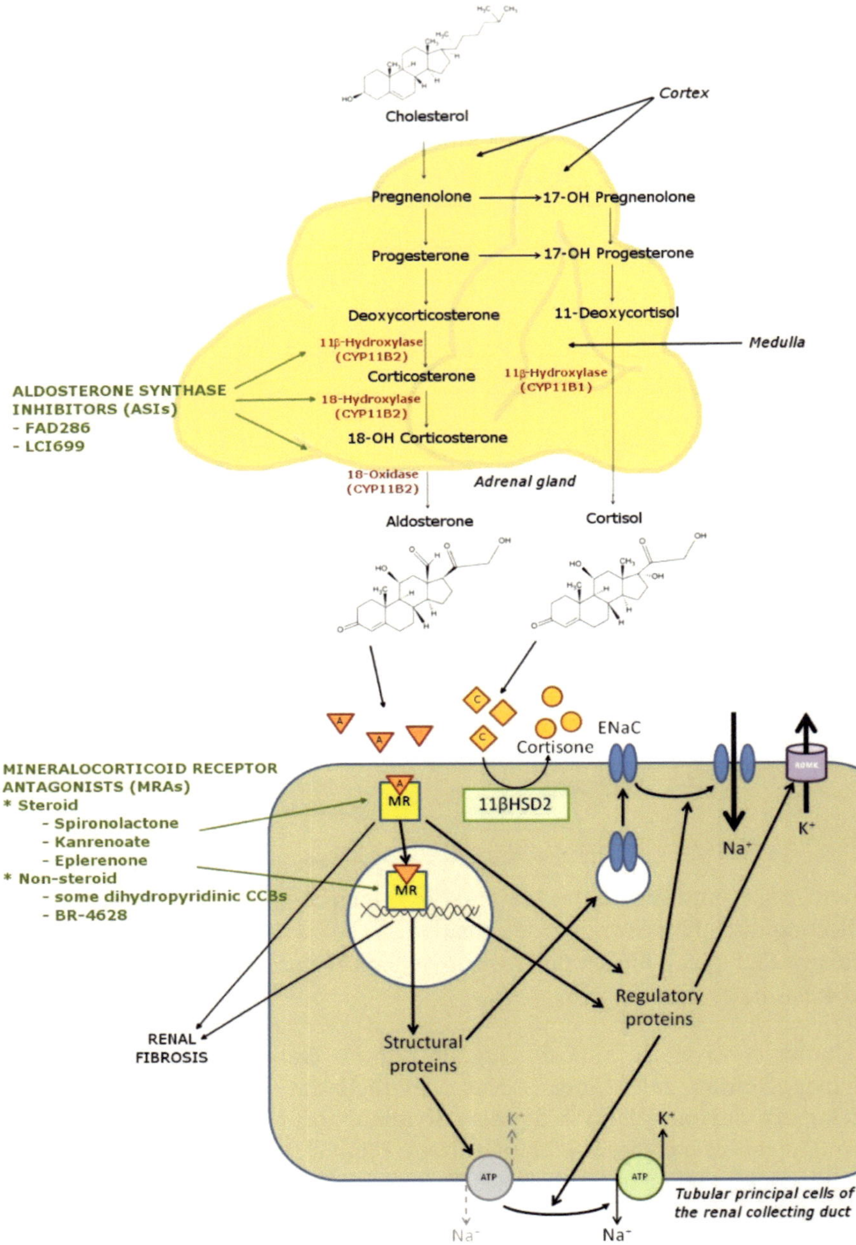

Fig. 3. Aldosterone (A) and cortisol (C) synthesis in the adrenal cortex and mechanisms of aldosterone action in the principal cells of the collecting duct. Aldosterone and cortisol originate from the metabolic conversion of cholesterol in the adrenal cortex. Finals steps of this conversion involve the cytochrome P450 enzymes CYP11B2 and CYP11B1 for the synthesis of aldosterone and cortisol, respectively. Aldosterone synthase inhibitors selectively block CYP11B2 and reduce aldosterone levels. In tubular cells, aldosterone activates the mineralocorticoid receptor and thereby induces structural and regulatory proteins that increase the activity of the epithelial sodium channel (ENaC), the renal outer

medullary potassium channel (ROMK), and the sodium/potassium ATPase pump. The net effect is sodium reabsorption in the bloodstream and potassium excretion in urine. Steroidal or non-steroidal mineralocorticoid receptor antagonists block the mineralocorticoid receptor activation by aldosterone. Inappropriate activation of mineralocorticoid receptors by cortisol is inhibited by its conversion to the receptor-inactive cortisone by the 11β-hydroxysteroid dehydrogenase (11βHSD2).

In vitro experiments have demonstrated that changes in the redox potential of cardiomyocytes by exposure to oxidized glutathione turn cortisol from being a receptor antagonist to an agonist. More recently, it has been demonstrated that aldosterone itself induces changes in the intracellular redox potential in diverse cell types through an activation of the NOX1 catalytic subunit of NAD(P)H oxidase. This aldosterone-dependent change in the redox potential is amplified by exposure to high concentrations of salt leading to increased production of ROS and thereby to cellular and tissue injury.

In fact, ROS are responsible for apoptosis of cardiomyocytes and for mesangial cell proliferation and matrix expansion in glomeruli of rats. In vascular tissues a slight increase in sodium concentration in the presence of aldosterone affects the biomechanical properties of the endothelial cells leading to cell swelling and cell stiffening (Figure 4). Both these effects are blunted by amiloride (a selective ENaC inhibitor) or spironolactone demonstrating the involvement of a mineralocorticoid receptor-dependent activation of ENaC pathway also in the vascular tissue (Figure 4). Furthermore, the analysis of gene expression profiling of vascular tissues demonstrated that, in the context of an enhanced oxidative stress, aldosterone can stimulate the expression of several pro-atherogenic genes and this expression can be inhibited by mineralocorticoid receptor antagonists.

Thus, in addition to the well-known effects of salt loading on epithelial swelling, vascular stiffening and blood pressure increase, some effects of salt loading might depend on mineralocorticoid receptor activation and reflect, in different tissues, impairment of 11β-HSD2 activity and/or increased oxidative stress, both mechanisms possibly leading to changes in the intracellular redox state. The distinction of these effects of salt from those generated at the tissue level by elevated aldosterone is complex and even genetic manipulations could not help in the understanding of their respective roles. In fact, both cardiac overexpression of the mineralocorticoid receptor and cardiac-specific induction of aldosterone production do not cause cardiac fibrosis, whereas fibrosis results from knockdown of the cardiac receptor by the use of antisense mRNA.

Although the use of mineralocorticoid receptor antagonists can inhibit or reduce aldosterone effects, several rapid actions of aldosterone on vascular tissue, such as regulation of vascular tone are, at least in part, independent of mineralocorticoid receptor blockade. Therefore, a mineralocorticoid receptor-independent pathway and the existence of a new aldosterone receptor have been hypothesized (Figure 4). Recently, it has been shown that in vascular smooth muscle aldosterone action is linked to a mineralocorticoid receptor-independent pathway that is mediated by the G protein coupled receptor (GPR30) (Figure 4). This pathway involves phosphatidylinositol 3-kinase (PI3K) and the extracellular signal-regulated kinase (ERK). These findings rise new questions on the role of aldosterone-related and mineralocorticoid receptor-independent pathways in causing tissue injury.

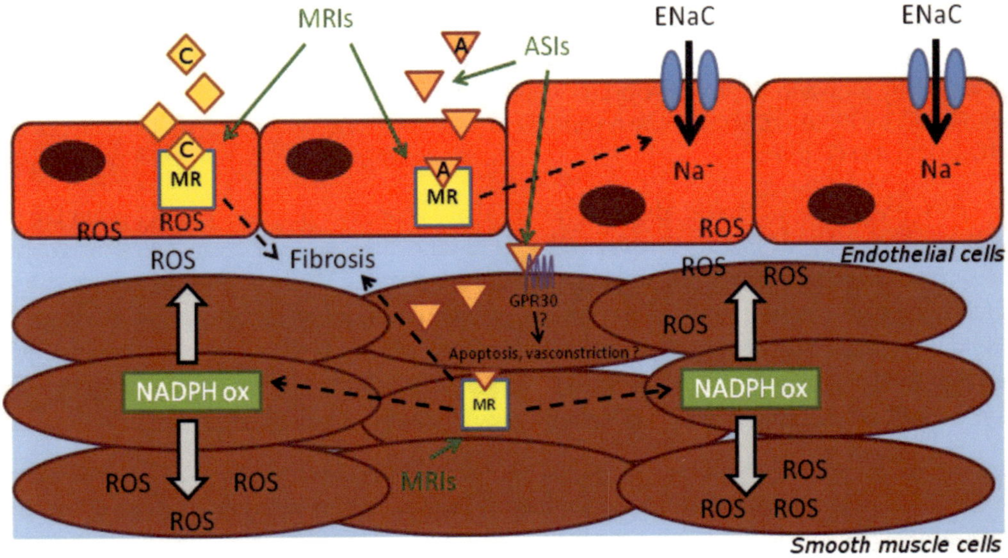

Fig. 4. Effect of aldosterone (A) on blood vessels. Aldosterone binds to mineralocorticoid receptors (MR) increasing generation of reactive oxygen species (ROS) and induces endothelial cell swelling and stiffening via a mineralocorticoid receptor-dependent pathway involving the NADPH oxidase and epithelial sodium channel, respectively. Both effects are blocked by mineralocorticoid receptor antagonists. Increased oxidative stress turns cortisol (C) to be an agonist rather than an antagonist of mineralocorticoid receptor. Aldosterone might exert its deleterious cardiovascular effects also through a mineralocorticoid receptor-independent pathway involving the G protein coupled receptor (GPR30) that can induce vascular smooth muscle cell apoptosis and inappropriate vasoconstriction. The pathophysiological role of these "non-genomic" effects of aldosterone needs to be further explored.

4. Spironolactone

Spironolactone (Figure 1) was synthesized in the Searle Laboratories in 1958 and its aldosterone blocking activity was discovered in 1959 (Cella et al., 1959). The molecule was approved for clinical use in 1962 and has been used for many decades in the treatment of primary aldosteronism, ascites associated with portal hypertension, and congestive heart failure. It has been used also for the treatment of primary hypertension (De Gasparo et al., 1987).

4.1 Metabolism

Spironolactone is a well-absorbed (approximately 65%), lipid-soluble, and highly protein bound steroidal aldosterone antagonist. It is largely metabolized in a hepatic first-pass with a high degree of enterohepatic cycling and a half-life of 1.6 hours, as such. In fact, spironolactone is transformed to either 7-thiomethylspirolactone or canrenone, two active metabolites that account for much of its pharmacological activity. Canrenone has a 20-hour half-life, but this is prolonged in patients with cardiac insufficiency. Spironolactone is also an inducer of microsomal drug metabolizing enzymes in the liver. The onset of action of spironolactone is slow, with a peak response that is reached approximately 48 hours after the first oral dose. Spironolactone is moderately more potent than eplerenone in blocking mineralocorticoid receptors. Spironolactone remains active when renal function is impaired because it reaches its site of action independent of glomerular filtration. This accounts for the risk of hyperkalemia observed in patients with chronic kidney disease and in patients with congestive heart failure and impaired renal function.

4.2 Dosing

The recommended oral dosing range of spironolactone is from 12.5 to 250 mg once or twice a day in primary hypertension and other disease conditions in which the use of this agent is indicated.

4.3 Clinical use

Spironolactone is a medication that has been used for more than 50 years to treat hypertension, edema, primary aldosteronism, and, more recent evidence indicates benefits also in patients with congestive heart failure and proteinuria.

Almost a decade ago, a landmark trial investigated the effects of spironolactone in patients with functional class III-IV systolic heart failure, showing a significant decrease in the mortality rate as compared to patients who received placebo on top of conventional treatment. The Randomized Aldactone Evaluation Study (RALES) (Pitt et al., 1999) was conducted in patients with New York Heart Association (NYHA) class III-IV heart failure who were treated with spironolactone. More recently, it has been suggested that the benefits of spironolactone in the context of cardiac failure are not restricted to patients with impaired systolic function and some studies have tested the effects of spironolactone in patients with heart failure and preserved systolic function (HFPSF). Edwards et al. reported improved diastolic function parameters with use of spironolactone in 112 patients with stage 2-3 chronic renal failure and HFPSF who were included in the Chronic Renal Impairment in Birmingham (CRIB II) study. In this study, the effects of spironolactone on left ventricular function and circulating markers of collagen turnover were compared with those of placebo. After 40 weeks, spironolactone improved significantly markers of left ventricular relaxation and attenuated significantly the increase in aminoterminal propeptide of type-III procollagen that was observed with placebo. This and other studies on HFPSF suggest a possible benefit of spironolactone also on this subtype of cardiac insufficiency. Notably, all these studies have employed doses of spironolactone (from 25 to 50 mg/day) that did not lower blood pressure suggesting that the cardioprotective effects of spironolactone occurs independent of the blood pressure-related hemodynamic load to the heart. Taken together, the findings obtained in the studies that have tested the effects of spironolactone in heart failure provide indirect evidence of untoward effect of aldosterone on the heart.

Many studies have reported a beneficial effect of blockers of the renin-angiotensin-aldosterone system in slowing down progression of renal disease, but the relative contributions of angiotensin II versus aldosterone have been dissociated only recently in animal studies. Clinical studies have supported the view that mineralocorticoid receptor blockade may exert an antialbuminuric effect in patients with proteinuria. In patients with diabetic nephropathy, it was shown that the antiproteinuric effect of angiotensin-converting enzyme (ACE) inhibitors reverts to baseline in patients who manifest aldosterone escape and that spironolactone combined with an ACE inhibitor results in an additional decrease in albuminuria (Sato et al., 2003). Also, spironolactone effectively reduced proteinuria in patients with idiopathic chronic glomerulonephritis previously treated with either ACE inhibitors or angiotensin receptor blockers (Bianchi et al., 2005). Another, more recent, study has shown that spironolactone added to an ACE inhibitor or an angiotensin receptor blocker reduces albuminuria in patients with type 2 diabetes and nephropathy. Collectively, these observations suggest that the mechanisms of the antialbuminuric effect of spironolactone are independent of blood pressure reduction and occur on top of those of other blockers of the renin-angiotensin system.

4.3.1 Essential hypertension

The anti-hypertensive effects of spironolactone have been overviewed in a recent meta-analysis that has included five cross-over studies and one randomized controlled trial with a total of 179 essential hypertensive patients that were followed from 4 to 8 weeks (Batterink et al., 2010). This meta-analysis showed that spironolactone decreases systolic and diastolic blood pressure by 20 and 7 mmHg, respectively, but this effect is reached with doses between 100 and 500 mg per day. With these doses, the risk of hyperkalemia is an important limitation and this is why use of spironolactone in the treatment of essential hypertension has been limited to combination with other types of diuretics. The dose of 25 mg/day did not change either systolic or diastolic blood pressure. None of the studies that were included in this meta-analysis reported results for hard endpoints such as mortality and major cardiovascular events. Therefore, at present there is no evidence that use of spironolactone decreases the risk of cardiovascular disease.

Despite the effects of spironolactone on blood pressure in essential hypertensive patients are modest and there is no demonstration that spironolactone protects from cardiovascular events, possible benefits on subclinical hypertensive organ damage that might be obtained even with the lower doses of the drug should be considered. Some small studies conducted in patients with hypertension-induced left ventricular hypertrophy have reported that addition of spironolactone to blockers of the renin-angiotensin system increases the effects on left ventricular mass reduction. The effects of an ACE-inhibitor alone or an ACE-inhibitor plus spironolactone (25 mg/day) on blood pressure and left ventricular mass changes were compared in essential hypertensive patients with left ventricular hypertrophy. Left ventricular mass index decreased in both treatment groups, but the extent of reduction was significantly greater in patients who were treated with the combination of the ACE-inhibitor and spironolactone. Similarly, the effects of candesartan (8 mg/day) alone or combined with spironolactone (25 mg/day) were tested in patients with hypertension and different patterns of left ventricular geometry. Changes in blood pressure did not differ between the two groups, whereas only the combination of candesartan and spironolactone decreased left ventricular mass with a change that was significant only in patients with concentric hypertrophy. In another study, 30 hypertensive patients with impaired diastolic function were randomized to receive either 25 mg/day of spironolactone or placebo for 6 months. Peak systolic strain and cyclic variation of integrated backscatter were improved by spironolactone with significant differences with patients treated with placebo. Thus, current evidence indicates that spironolactone could have a considerable place in the treatment of essential hypertensive patients with left ventricular hypertrophy and/or diastolic dysfunction.

4.3.2 Resistant hypertension

Several clinical case reports suggested that spironolactone can be useful in the treatment of resistant hypertension and, in particular, in hypertension associated to obesity or obstructive sleep apnea syndrome. One controlled and several non-controlled studies have confirmed that addition of 25-50 mg of spironolactone to current treatment effectively reduces blood pressure in patients with resistant hypertension. In the ASPIRANT trial, 117 patients with resistant hypertension were randomized to treatment with spironolactone or placebo in a double-blind protocol. The trial was prematurely stopped after the first interim analysis because of a significant reduction of systolic blood pressure in patients taking spironolactone as compared to those taking placebo. Notably, the average BMI of the study population in this trial was 32.3 clearly indicating that patients were either obese or overweight. In the prospective, uncontrolled study of Souza et al., 175 patients with resistant hypertension were treated with 25-100 mg/day of spironolactone and, after a median interval of 7 months, 24-hour systolic and diastolic blood pressure decreased by 16 mm Hg and 9 mm Hg, respectively. The baseline characteristics of these patients showed again that they were either overweight or obese and had high prevalence of diabetes, dyslipidemia, left ventricular hypertrophy, and previous cardiovascular diseases. In the ASCOT-BPLA trial, patients who took spironolactone as fourth line therapy because of resistant hypertension were analyzed retrospectively. In these patients, spironolactone at a median dose of 25 mg/day significantly reduced blood pressure by 21.9/9.5 mm. Even in this study, patients with resistant hypertension had significantly higher body mass index, systolic blood pressure, and prevalence of diabetes and left ventricular hypertrophy than patients who were not resistant to treatment. Very similar results were reported in other studies conducted on patients of different geographical areas.

The beneficial effect of spironolactone in patients with resistant hypertension is currently unexplained, although this effect suggests a substantial contribution of aldosterone to maintenance of increased blood pressure despite of treatment. Inappropriate secretion of aldosterone has been reported in hypertensive patients with associated obesity and/or obstructive sleep apnea syndrome. Also, it is well known that aldosterone can escape the inhibitory effects of renin-angiotensin system blockers in patients treated with these drugs, thereby leading to a form of hypertension that is largely aldosterone-dependent. Finally, it cannot be excluded that, at least in some cases, resistance to antihypertensive treatment hides a mild form of primary aldosteronism.

4.3.3 Primary aldosteronism

Spironolactone is the drug of choice in the medical treatment of primary aldosteronism in which hypertension is due to an excessive aldosterone secretion from the adrenal gland. In this clinical setting, spironolactone reduces blood pressure, corrects hypokalemia, and reverts cardiac and renal abnormalities as it has been reviewed recently. This was demonstrated in long-term follow-up studies in which treatment with spironolactone reduced cardiovascular and renal events and decreased left ventricular mass and urinary protein excretion in patients with primary aldosteronism (Sechi et al., 2010).

Cardiovascular outcomes were compared in 108 patients with essential hypertension and in 54 patients with primary aldosteronism who were comparable for demographic variables and had comparable risk factors, but greater retrospective incidence of coronary artery disease, cerebrovascular events, and sustained arrhythmias (Catena et al. 2008). Patients were followed for an average of 7.4 years after surgical removal of an adrenal adenoma or treatment with spironolactone, with a combined end point including myocardial infarction, stroke, any type of revascularization procedure, and sustained arrhythmias. During follow-up, blood pressure was comparable in the primary aldosteronism and essential hypertension group, and 10 patients in the former group and 19 in the latter group reached the end point. Actuarial analysis of patients treated with surgery vs. spironolactone did not reveal significant difference in the occurrence of the combined end point. In the same cohort of patients, the outcomes of renal function were investigated by measuring the rates of change of glomerular filtration and albuminuria (Sechi et al., 2006). After an initial decline in creatinine clearance, due to correction of the aldosterone-induced intrarenal hemodynamic adaptation, subsequent decrease of glomerular filtration in patients with primary aldosteronism and essential hypertension were comparable. Urinary albumin losses did not differ between patients with primary aldosteronism and essential hypertension during follow-up. Evaluation of renal outcomes in patients with primary aldosteronism who were treated with surgery or spironolactone did not reveal significant difference. These two studies clearly demonstrate that spironolactone has the same therapeutic value as surgery in the treatment of primary aldosteronism and in the prevention of cardiovascular and renal complications.

In addition to excess cardiovascular and renal events as compared to matched patients with essential hypertension, patients with primary aldosteronism are characterized by cardiac, renal, and metabolic subclinical structural and functional abnormalities (Rossi et al., 2008). A number of cross-sectional cardiac ultrasound studies have reported an excess increase of left ventricular mass in patients with primary aldosteronism as compared to other types of hypertensive disease. In a 7-year echocardiographic study it was demonstrated that patients with primary aldosteronism treated with either surgery or spironolactone have significant and comparable decrease of left ventricular mass, although decrease is significant within the first year only after adrenalectomy (Catena et al., 2007). We have already mentioned the effects of spironolactone on correction of albuminuria. These effects are at least in part related to reversal of an intrarenal hemodynamic adaptation to aldosterone excess with a vasodilatory response that has been demonstrated with intrarenal echo-Doppler examination (Sechi et al., 2009).

5. Canrenoate

Canrenone (Figure 1) is one of the two metabolites of spironolactone. It is administered orally as a potassium salt (potassium canrenoate) that is mineralocorticoid receptor-inactive, but it is rapidly transformed to canrenone. Canrenone is water soluble, and this characteristic permits intravenous administration when a rapid effect is desired.

Potassium canrenoate exerts its hypotensive effect approximately one week after the starting dose. Both canrenone and canrenoate are rapidly absorbed (approximately 80%) after oral administration. Both agents have important plasma protein binding (approximately 90%) with small volumes of distribution.

6. Eplerenone

Eplerenone (Figure 1) has been synthesized in the attempt to obtain a more selective inhibition of the mineralocorticoid receptors to overcome the side effects due to cross-reaction of spironolactone and canrenone with androgen receptors. It was synthesized in the

Ciba-Geigy laboratories in the mid-80s and was approved in the United States for clinical use in arterial hypertension in 2002.

6.1 Pharmacology

Eplerenone was synthesized by replacing the 17-thioacetyl group with a carbomethoxy group in the molecule of spironolactone (Figure 1). The critical feature in the eplerenone molecule however, conferring enhanced mineralocorticoid receptor selectivity is the presence of the epoxide group in the lactone ring. The activity of eplerenone in vitro was assessed in vitro using recombinant steroid receptors. The potency of eplerenone at other steroid receptors was significantly reduced and, unlike previous aldosterone blockers, eplerenone possesses very low activity on the androgen, progesterone, and glucocorticoid receptors.

Oral bioavailability is approximately 95% and meals have no effect on the extent of absorption. Eplerenone does not undergo relevant metabolic first-pass in the liver neither it induces cytochrome P450 activity, although interactions with drugs that are metabolized by cytochrome P450 are not excluded. The two main metabolites of eplerenone (6β-OH eplerenone and open lactone ring) are both mineralocorticoid receptor-inactive. The plasma half-life of eplerenone is approximately 5 hours.

The recommended oral dosing range for eplerenone is from 50 to 100 mg once or twice daily in essential hypertension. No correlations between eplerenone disposal and renal function have been found.

6.2 Clinical use

Eplerenone has come into the clinical arena in the last decade and has been employed to lower blood pressure in essential hypertensive patients. Similar to spironolactone, recent studies have reported beneficial effects of eplerenone in congestive heart failure and renal disease with proteinuria. The Eplerenone Post-Acute Myocardial Infarction Heart Failure Efficacy and Survival Study (EPHESUS) (Pitt et al. 2003) investigated the effects of eplerenone in post-myocardial infarction patients with severely impaired left ventricular function, showing a significant decrease in the mortality rate as compared to patients who received placebo on top of conventional treatment. Recently, these observations have been extended to patients with milder degrees of cardiac dysfunction in the Eplerenone in Mild Patients Hospitalization and Survival Study in Heart Failure (EMPHASIS-HF) (Zannad et al., 2011) study. In this study, 2737 patients with NYHA class II cardiac insufficiency and left ventricular ejection fraction of less than 35% were randomized to receive either eplerenone or placebo in addition to conventional treatment. This trial ended prematurely after a median follow-up of 21 months because the composite endpoint of cardiovascular death and hospitalization for heart failure were significantly less frequent in patients who were treated with eplerenone. Thus, eplerenone seems to be beneficial even at the early stages of systolic cardiac failure.

As for spironolactone, the possibility that eplerenone may result beneficial also in patients with HFPSF has been investigated. Forty-four elderly patients with heart failure and left ventricular ejection fraction of more than 45% were randomized to conventional treatment with or without eplerenone and left ventricular function was reassessed with conventional echocardiography and tissue Doppler imaging at 6 and 12 months. In patients who were treated with eplerenone, deceleration time had a significantly greater decrease than in patients on conventional treatment and, after 12 months, the eplerenone-induced improvement of diastolic function was associated with a significantly slower increase in plasma procollagen levels. Both studies on systolic and diastolic heart failure were conducted with doses of eplerenone (from 25 to 50 mg/day) that did not lower blood pressure.

Consistent with previous findings using spironolactone, eplerenone has been demonstrated to confer renal protection independent of its effects on blood pressure. Eplerenone was administered in doses of 50 and 100 mg/day to patients with type 2 diabetes and albuminuria who were already treated with an ACE inhibitor. After 4, 8, and 12 weeks, both doses of eplerenone induced significant reduction of urinary protein losses as compared to placebo, whereas blood pressure levels did not differ during follow-up. Effects of the two doses of eplerenone were comparable (Epstein, 2003).

6.2.1 Essential hypertension

Eplerenone has been repeatedly tested in patients with mild to moderate essential hypertension. One uncontrolled open-label study and many randomized controlled trials have documented the antihypertensive effect of eplerenone when compared to either placebo or other classes of antihypertensive agents. Controlled studies have compared the blood pressure lowering effects of eplerenone at doses comprised form 50 to 400 mg/day with those of either placebo, enalapril, losartan, amlodipine, or spironolactone. In these studies, follow-up duration was from 2 to 14 months. In all studies, eplerenone was more effective than placebo in reducing blood pressure, in two studies it was more potent than losartan, and in the remaining studies the hypotensive effects were comparable to those of enalapril, amlodipine, and spironolactone. Similar to spironolactone, none of these studies reported results for hard cardiovascular endpoints including mortality and major cardiovascular events and therefore there is no evidence that eplerenone improves cardiovascular outcomes in hypertensive patients.

Eplerenone has been demonstrated to be beneficial also on hypertension-related subclinical organ damage. In the 4-E Left Ventricular Hypertrophy Study, regression of left ventricular hypertrophy was compared in essential hypertensive patients who were treated with eplerenone, enalapril, or their combination for 9 months. Left ventricular mass index decreased significantly and comparably in patients treated with eplerenone or enalapril, whereas the combination of the two agents showed additive effects on left ventricular mass reduction. In other studies, eplerenone was reported to be more effective than amlodipine, enalapril, or losartan in decreasing urinary albumin excretion.

Despite eplerenone has a satisfactory tolerability and safety profile even at the highest doses that have been clinically tested (200 mg/day), its effects on blood pressure in essential hypertension and primary aldosteronism are inferior to those of spironolactone.

7. Epithelial sodium channel blockers

ENaC blockers are potassium-sparing compounds with weak diuretic properties. Both amiloride and triamterene are treatment of choice in the Liddle syndrome, but are relatively uneffective in essential hypertension when used as monotherapy and can be useful when used in combination with other types of diuretics that cause hypokalemia such as thiazides and loop diuretics.

No studies have evaluated the effects of ENaC blockers in monotherapy in patients with essential hypertension. Four studies with amiloride and 2 studies with triamterene have evaluated the dose-related blood pressure efficacy of these drugs when added, as a second antihypertensive agent, to hydrochlorothiazide or chlorthalidone (Heran et al., 2010).

7.1 Amiloride

Amiloride is a selective blocker of the ENaC. It is actively secreted by cationic carriers in the proximal tubule, reaching its active site at the distal tubule. At this level, amiloride indirectly antagonizes the effects of aldosterone on sodium-potassium exchange leading to increased sodium excretion with relative potassium retention. Amiloride is cleared by the kidney and can accumulate in patients with impaired renal function. Therefore, the dosage should be reduced when the glomerular filtration rate is below 50 ml/min.

No studies have evaluated amiloride as monotherapy in patients with essential hypertension. Amiloride is administered in patients with essential hypertension usually in combination with thiazide diuretics. Amiloride can also be used in patients with primary aldosteronism when spironolactone is not tolerated. Although studies that have tested amiloride as an antihypertensive agents have reported good tolerability, particular caution is required in patients with renal failure or in patients treated with blockers of the renin-angiotensin system because of the risk of hyperkalemia.

Data on use of amiloride (from 2.5 to 5 mg/day) in combination with hydrochlorothiazide are insufficient to demonstrate a significant difference between treatment with the combination and hydrochlorothiazide alone. Therefore current evidence does not support any effect of low doses of amiloride on blood pressure. No trials evaluating doses of amiloride higher than 5 mg/day have been performed and therefore a dose-response relationship with the hypotensive effect can not be demonstrated. No effects of amiloride on pulse pressure or blood pressure variability could be demonstrated in the studies that have employed this agent in the treatment of hypertension.

There are no appropriately designed studies that have tested the effects of amiloride in other disease conditions. In primary aldosteronism experiences are mainly anedoctal and the doses of this drug to use in this context have never been defined with precision. No studies have been performed to test the effects of amiloride on subclinical hypertensive organ damage, heart failure, and proteinuria.

7.2 Triamterene

Similar to amiloride, triamterene blocks the ENaC in the distal tubular site of the nephron. Triamterene is incompletely absorbed and is transformed to a sulphate-conjugated metabolite. It gains access to the tubular lumen via a cationic transporter in the proximal tubule. Both triamterene and its metabolite accumulate in patients with renal failure. When used alone, triamterene has little effect on blood pressure. Therefore it is usually employed in combination to compensate for the hypokalemic effects of other diuretics.

No studies have evaluated triamterene as monotherapy in patients with essential hypertension. Data on use of triamterene (50 mg/day) in combination with chlorthalidone are insufficient to demonstrate a significant difference between treatment with the combination and chlorthalidone alone. Therefore current evidence does not support any effect of low doses of triamterene on blood pressure. No data are currently available on the effects on blood pressure of higher doses of triamterene and therefore a dose-response relationship with the hypotensive effect can not be demonstrated. No effects of triamterene on pulse pressure or blood pressure variability could be demonstrated in the studies that have employed this agent in the treatment of hypertension. Tolerability and safety profile of triamterene in the studies that have tested this drug were acceptable.

There are no studies that have tested the effects of triamterene in other disease conditions. In primary aldosteronism experiences are mainly anedoctal and the doses of this drug that should be used in this endocrine disorder have never been specifically defined. No studies have been conducted to investigate the effects of triamterene on subclinical hypertensive organ damage, heart failure, and proteinuria.

8. New aldosterone blockers

Promising results with mineralocorticoid receptor antagonists in the treatment of hypertension and prevention of hypertension-related organ damage have prompted the search and possible development of new aldosterone antagonists. Search has followed two main strategies: the first has consisted in the development of non-steroidal antagonists that could overcome the side effects of spironolactone and canrenoate without losing the pharmacological properties of these compounds; the second has aimed at developing drugs that inhibit aldosterone biosynthesis and has resulted in the generation of aldosterone synthase direct inhibitors.

8.1 Non steroidal mineralocorticoid receptor antagonists

The first strategy moved its initial steps from the demonstration that some dyhydropyridine calcium-channel blockers (CCBs) exerts also a mineralocorticoid receptor antagonist activity. Researchers in the Pfizer® laboratories reported that nimodipine, felodipine, and nitrendipine block aldosterone-induced receptor activation by competing with aldosterone binding to the receptor "ligand binding domain". The affinity of dihydropyridines for the receptor binding domain is lower than for the L-type calcium channels, indicating that inhibition of mineralocorticoid receptor activity is independent of the effects on calcium channels. The efficacy of dyihydropyridines as mineralocorticoid receptor antagonist is comparable to that of eplerenone, whereas non-dihydropyridine CCBs such as verapamil and diltiazem do not have any inhibitory activity.

8.2 Aldosterone synthase inhibitors

The other new class of anti-aldosterone agents includes the selective aldosterone-synthase inhibitors. Aldosterone synthase or CYP11B2 is an enzyme of the cytochrome P450 family with steroid 18-hydroxylase and 18-oxidase properties. It catalyzes the formation of aldosterone from 11-deoxycorticosterone within the zona glomerulosa in the adrenal cortex (Figure 3). CYP11B2 deficiency in humans is characterized by a low/absent aldosterone synthesis in the adrenal cortex, high plasma renin activity and is responsible for a sodium-wasting phenotype associated with retarded growth. Conversely, enhanced activation of CYP11B2 as it is supposed to occur in the polymorphism 344C/T, is associated with increased left ventricular mass and greater risk to develop hypertension. Since CYP11B2 activity is the limiting biochemical step in aldosterone synthesis, its selective inhibition is a good target for prevention of aldosterone untoward effects mediated by both mineralocorticoid receptor-dependent and mineralocorticoid receptor-independent pathways.

At present, only two compounds (both synthesized by Novartis®) with selective CYP11B2 inhibitory properties have been tested in animal models and, very recently, in the clinical setting. FAD286 is the D-enantiomer of the fadrozole, an aromatase inhibitor developed to treat advanced breast cancer, that reduces aldosterone levels and increases plasma renin activity in rats fed with either low or high sodium diet. In a transgenic rat model of secondary hypertension in which the angiotensinogen gene is overexpressed and circulating angiotensin II levels are increased, oral administration of FAD286 has reduced mortality by 4 times. In transgenic rats treated with FAD286, cardiac hypertrophy, albuminuria, and histologic evidence of glomerular damage were less frequent than in control animals. Despite very minor effects of FAD286 on blood pressure, its effects on organ damage were comparable to those of the angiotensin receptor blocker, losartan.

Following promising preclinical results, the first aldosterone synthase inhibitor, LCI699, was tested in two phase-II clinical trials. LCI699 is similar in structure to FAD286 and it has been developed for human use. LCI699 was administered to 14 patients affected by primary aldosteronism and effects were compared to those of placebo. After 2 weeks of treatment, there was a dose-dependent decrease in plasma aldosterone and an increase in 11-deoxycorticosterone, potassium, and adrenocorticotropin levels. Treatment induced mild reduction of 24-h ambulatory systolic blood pressure by (4.1 mm Hg) after 4 weeks. More recently, Calhoun et al. have published the first randomized, double-blind, placebo controlled phase-II trial with LCI699 that was conducted in 524 patients with essential hypertension. In this trial different doses of LCI699 have reduced 24-h ambulatory systolic blood pressure, but only the highest dose has reduced also diastolic blood pressure.

9. Acknowledgments

This work was supported by a research grant of the Pier Silverio Nassimbeni Foundation.

10. References

Batterink, J. et al. (2010). Spironolactone for hypertension. *Cochrane Database of Systematic Reviews,* Issue.1, CD008169

Bianchi, S., Bigazzi, R. & Campese, V.M. (2005). Antagonists of aldosterone and proteinuria in patients with CKD: an uncontrolled pilot study. *American Journal of Kidney Diseases,* Vol.46, pp. 45-51, PMID 15983956

Catena, C. et al. (2007). Long-term cardiac effects of adrenalectomy or mineralocorticoid antagonists in patients with primary aldosteronism. *Hypertension,* Vol.50, pp. 911-918, PMID 17893375

Catena, C. et al. (2008). Cardiovascular outcomes in patients with primary aldosteronism after treatment. *Archives of Internal Medicine,* Vol.168, pp. 80-85, PMID 18195199

Cella, J., Brown, E.A. & Burtner, R.R. (1959). Steroidal aldosterone blockers. *Journal of Organic Chemistry,*Vol.24, pp. 743-748

De Gasparo, M. et al. (1987) Three new epoxy-spironolactone derivatives: characterization in vivo and in vitro. *Journal of Pharmacology and Experimental Therapeutics,* Vol.240, pp. 650-656, PMID 2949071

Epstein, M. (2003). Aldosterone receptor blockade and the role of eplerenone: evolving perspectives. *Nephrology Dialysis Transplantation,* Vol.18: pp. 1984-1992, PMID 13679471

Garthwaite, S.M. & McMahon E.G. (2004). The evolution of aldosterone antagonists. *Molecular and CellularEndocrinology,* Vol.217, pp. 27-31, PMID 15134797

Heran, B.S. et al. (2010). Blood pressure lowering efficacy of potassium-sparing diuretics (that block the epithelial sodium channel) for primary hypertension. *Cochrane Database of Systematic Reviews,* Issue.1, CD008167

Marney, A.M. & Brown, N. J. (2007) Aldosterone and end-organ damage. *Clinical Science,* Vol.113, pp. 267-278, PMID17683282

Pitt, B. et al. (1999).The effect of spironolactone on morbidity and mortality in patients with severe heart failure. Randomized Aldactone Evaluation Study Investigators. *The New England Journal of Medicine,* Vol.341, pp. 709-717, PMID 10471456

Pitt, B. et al. (2003). Eplerenone, a selective aldosterone blocker, in patients with left ventricular dysfunction after myocardial infarction. *The New England Journal of Medicine,* Vol.348, pp. 1309-1321, PMID 12668699

Prospective Studies Collaboration. (2002). Age-specific relevance of usual blood pressure to vascular mortality: a meta-analysis of individual data for one million adults in 61 prospective studies. *The Lancet,* Vol.360, pp. 1903–1913, PMID 12493255

Rossi, G.P. et al. (2008). Primary aldosteronism: cardiovascular, renal and metabolic implications. *Trends in Endocrinology and Metabolism,* Vol.19, pp. 88–90, PMID 18314347

Sato, A. et al. (2003). Effectiveness of aldosterone blockade in patients with diabetic nephropathy. *Hypertension,*Vol41, pp. 64-68, PMID 12511531

Sechi, L.A. et al. (2006). Long-term renal outcomes in patients with primary aldosteronism. *JAMA,* Vol.295, pp. 2638-2645, PMID 16772627

Sechi, L.A. et al. (2009). Intrarenal hemodynamics in primary aldosteronism before and after treatment. *Journal of Clinical Endocrinology and Metabolism,* Vol.94, pp. 1191-1197, PMID 19141581

Sechi, L.A. et al. (2010). Cardiovascular and renal damage in primary aldosteronism: outcomes after treatment. *American Journal of Hypertension,* Vol.23, pp. 1253-1260, PMID 20706195

The Task Force for the Management of Arterial Hypertension of the European Society of Hypertension (ESH) and of the European Society of Cardiology (ESC). (2007). 2007 Guidelines for the Management of Arterial Hypertension. *Journal of Hypertension,* Vol.25, pp. 1105-1187, PMID 17762635

Wolf-Maier, K. et al. (2003). Hypertension prevalence and blood pressure levels in 6 European countries, Canada, and the United States. *Journal of the American Medical Association,* Vol.289, pp. 2363–2369, PMID 12746359

Zannad, F. et al. (2011). Eplerenone in patients with systolic heart failure and mild symptoms. *The New England Journal of Medicine,* Vol.364: pp. 11-21, PMID 21073363

5

Hypertension and Renin-Angiotensin System

Roberto de Barros Silva
Pharmaceutical Sciences Faculty of Ribeirao Preto FCFRP/USP, São Paulo, Brazil

1. Introduction

The renin-angiotensin system (RAS) participates in numerous biological activities. Among these is the pathophysiological mechanisms of hypertension, congestive heart failure, myocardial infarction, diabetic nephropathy and inflammatory disorders. These pleiotropic effects led to the development of new therapeutic approaches to inhibit the actions of this system. This chapter aims to relate the inflammatory process with the RAS thus focusing on the effects of antihypertensive drugs in the therapeutic and / or prevention of pathophysiological conditions. Also discussed in this chapter also the pharmacodynamic of ACE inhibitors, ARB inhibitors and Direct Renin Inhibitors, as well as a review of the RAS.

For a better knowledge of the system, it is necessary to first discuss the history of RAS components and focusing on general biochemistry, cell biology in its overall effects.

2. Renin-angiotensin system

The RAS is classically known as a circulatory system or hormone that regulates blood pressure and homeostasis of electrolytes and fluids. This classic study is originated from 1898 when Tiergersted and Bergman found that the kidney contained a pressor substance, through non-purified salt extracts, which was called renin. This discovery came only to attract attention with Goldblatt et al in the twentieth century in 1934 when they demonstrated that the constriction of the renal arteries producing persistent hypertension in dogs due to reduction in vascular area with a consequent increase in strength and blood pressure (Goldman and Gilman, 2007). Six years later he declared that the renin was actually a protein that acted on a substrate in plasma. The name of this substrate for 20 years was controversial, as two groups of researchers, one from Argentina and other U.S. called them differently. The first group was called the substrate of *hipertensin* and the second *angiotonin* until these names were changed to *angiotensin*, the true pressor material. The precursor of this peptide was called angiotensinogen. Therefore, the time had an idea this simplified system, Figure 1.

In the 50's has been identified two forms of angiotensin, respectively called of angiotensin I and II. The first would be a chain of 10 peptides, hence the term decapeptide. In contrast, the second would be formed by cleavage of two peptides of angiotensin I to form an octapeptide. This cleavage occurs through the participation of an enzyme located on the luminal surface of endothelial cells of vascular system known as Angiotensin Converting

Enzyme (ACE). In the overview of the peptide angiotensin II is more active, that is, angiotensin II that has the main vasoconstrictor effect. Thus by mid-50, the overall picture of this system was extended by both the description of the two angiotensins, and by the observation that this system RAS concurrently regulated secretion of aldosterone. Based on this knowledge that was acquired, the 70 and 80 was an improvement on the findings of these polypeptides that interfere with components of the RAS, is directly inhibiting the release of renin, or ACE, and angiotensin receptor antagonists. Anyway, these findings allow to the present day an increase in quality of life, these compounds being the main drug involved in the treatment of hypertension, congestive heart failure, diabetic nephropathy, myocardial infarction, more recent studies show the effects of these in inflammatory disorders. To understand this 'fine' relationship between RAS and inflammatory process, it is to reading the components of this system.

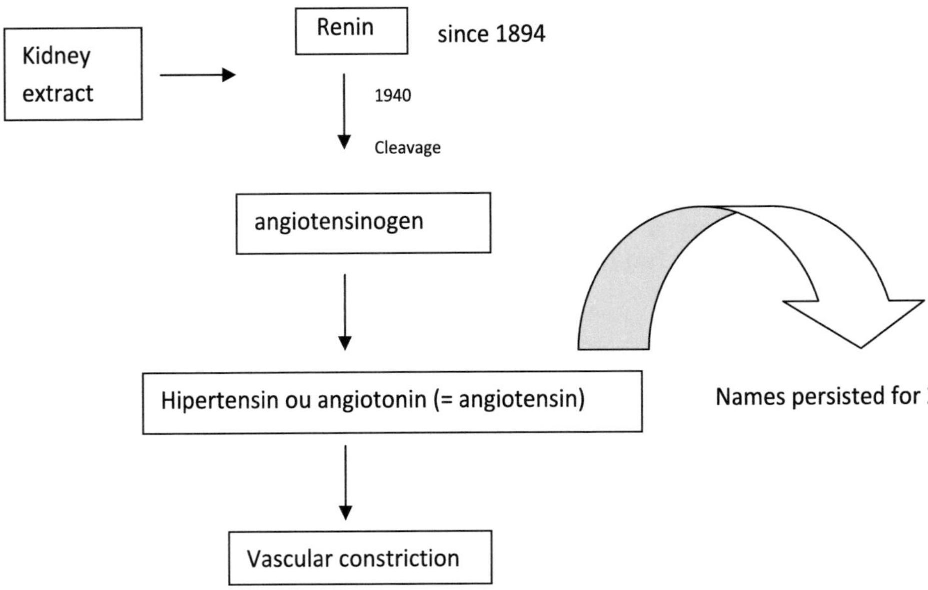

Fig. 1. Diagram showing the evolution in a simplified manner on the physiology of RAS. [Figure made by Barros, RS - 2011].

3. Renin angiotensin system components

Renin: It is the major protease able of determining the rate of production of angiotensin II. Renin is produced, stored and secreted in so-called juxtaglomerular cells, cells that are circulating in the renal artery, present in the afferent arterioles, ie, the infiltrating *glomerulus* in promoting renal perfusion in this region. The release of renin is done through a process called as exocytosis. The main substrate of this aspartyl protease is an α2 - globulin stock, ie, angiotensinogen that is secreted by hepatocytes. Regardless, the renin, which cleaves peptide bonds aminoterminal tail of the angiotensinogen (Leucyl-leucine in mice and rats) and (Leucine-valine in humans), leading to angiotensin I, is an active renin. Thus the synthesis of this protease is done in stages. The active form that contains 340 amino acids. It is synthesized as a pre-pro-enzyme with 406 amino acid residues, soon after, this precursor is processed and thus generates a pro-renin, which is a more mature, but no activity. Soon after this process pro-renin is activated by an enzyme not yet characterized, but cleaves 43 amino acids of the aminoterminal tail, thereby generating active renin. The secretion of renin by the juxtaglomerular cells (CJG) is controlled mainly by three ways: two act locally in the kidney and third acts indirectly through the CNS that releases norepinephrine from noradrenergic nerves of the kidney. The macula densa is a mechanism that controls the release of renin. It is a complex mechanism that relies on receptors, cyclic adenosine monophosphate (cAMP) and also through prostaglandins. In general, the macula densa is located adjacent to the CJG and is composed of columnar epithelial cells. When any change occurs in the flow of NaCl present in the macula densa cells release chemical signals that the CJG will inhibit or stimulate renin in the event of an increase or reduction of NaCl respectively. These signals via macula is mediated by both adenosine and prostaglandin by the first of which operates in the increase of NaCl and the second reduction. Regardless of which protein will act (adenosine or prostaglandin), the fact is that the answer to these is through the binding of these G protein coupled receptors, which will promote a signal dependent on the cellular second messenger (cAMP). Thus while acting within the A1 adenosine receptor adenosine inhibits renin release, while the prostaglandin stimulates.

The second mechanism that controls the release of renin is intrarenal baroreceptor pathway. This mechanism is regulated by raising and lowering blood pressure in pre-glomerular vessels, and thus are regulated by mechanical phenomenon. This mechanical modulation causes CJG inhibit or stimulate the release of renin. Moreover, the increase or reduction in renal perfusion pressure may inhibit the release or renal prostaglandin which act in part via the intrarenal baroreceptor.

Finally, the third mechanism is called via the beta-adrenergic receptors. In this case, regulation occurs via the CNS. After the release and action of this neurotransmitter norepinephrine from postganglionic sympathetic nerves occurs when it binds to beta-adrenergic receptors stimulating the sympathetic pathway and consequently the secretion of renin by CJG.

These three mechanisms of regulation of renin secretion are involved in a physiological network, explained below:

1. The increased release of renin leads to increased release of angiotensin II. This in turn binds to AT1 receptors in the CJG. This binding leads to inhibition of renin secretion in a mechanism known as short feedback loop.
2. In addition to angiotensin II also leads to an increase in blood pressure by binding these AT1 receptors. In increased pressure leads to a reduction in renin secretion through the action of high pressure baroreceptors, increased pressure from pre-glomerular vessels and reduced pressure natriuresis (drop in reabsorption of NaCl). This mechanism of reduction of renin secretion via increased blood pressure arising from the effects of angiotensin II is known as negative feedback loop long.

Angiotensionogen: It is important to a globular protein, has a (MW = 55,000 to 60,000) and is the main substrate of renin. The angiotensinogen is synthesized in the liver, although it may have also made their transcription in adipose tissue in the CNS and kidney. There is a very close relationship between the synthesis and secretion of angiotensinogen by stimuli such as inflammation, insulin, estrogens, glucocorticoids, thyroid hormone and angiotensin II, ie, all these stimuli increase the synthesis and secretion of dodecahydrate peptide. There is a strong relationship between the amount of circulating *angiotensinogen* in plasma and increased blood pressure, so the use of oral contraceptives containing estrogen lead to an increase in serum angiotensinogen, thereby resulting in an elevation of blood pressure. At this point becomes more clear also the strong relationship with the inflammatory process. We have seen that directly interferes with the prostaglandin release of renin, ie, prostaglandins increase the secretion of this hormone by binding to adenosine receptors.

Angiotensin Converting Enzyme (ACE): ACE is a glycoprotein ecto-enzyme and that in addition to cleaving angiotensin I to angiotensin II forming this ecto-enzyme can also inactivate bradykinin, because ACE is very nonspecific and can cleave dipeptide units with many amino acid substrate. Therefore, the ACE inhibitors such as captopril and lisinopril, for example, are able to increase bradykinin and reduce angiotensin II. The rapid in vivo conversion of angiotensin I to II occurs through the action of ACE that is present on the luminal surface of endothelial cells throughout the vascular system. In addition to these effects of ACE some studies show the existence of a carboxypeptidase-related enzyme called ACE2 is capable of cleaving angiotensin I into (angiotensin 1-9) and angiotensin II (angiotensin 1-7). This enzyme is not inhibited by classic ACE inhibitors. Its physiological importance is not yet clear.

4. The renin-angiotensin system and its relationship with pathophisiology hypertension

The pathophysiology of hypertension is defined as a lasting elevation of blood pressure to ≥ 140/90 mmHg, as this procedure was used because most individuals with this pressure range belong to risk group cardiovascular disease and hypertension arising from the medical attention they deserve. This disease is like the most common cardiovascular disease and its prevalence increases with age.

The RAS participates as a key player in regulating blood pressure in both long and short term. This happens because the increase, even in modest concentrations of angiotensin II leads to an acute elevation of blood pressure. To get an idea in terms of values to angiotensin II is about 40 times more potent than norepinephrine and effective concentration (EC50) to angiotensin II acute elevation of blood pressure is approximately 0.3 nmol / l. In the presence of angiotensin II administered intravenously pressure rises in a few seconds and after a few minutes this reduces the normal rate. This effect is known as immediate pressor response is due to a rapid increase in total peripheral resistance. This increased resistance is a response that maintains blood pressure in the presence of an acute hypotensive response. Although the direct effects of angiotensin II on cardiac contractility and heart rate indirect in the rapid rise in blood pressure leads to activation of the baroreceptor reflex, and in a negative feedback, this occurs with the reduction of sympathetic tone and increase vagal tone.

On the other hand, there is a slow pressor response, which also occurs by the action of angiotensin II. Response to this pressure is stabilized for a long time. This slow pressor response is most likely due to reduced renal excretion function, causing an increase in fluid retention and salt and, with increasing pressure quently. Associated with these renal effects, angiotensin II in this response also induces the synthesis of endothelin-1 and superoxide anion, which can contribute to this type of slow pressor response. Other classical effects of angiotensin II on the pathophysiology of hypertension is the morphological alteration of the cardiovascular system, causing hypertrophy of cardiac and vascular cells, and increase the synthesis and deposition of collagen by cardiac fibroblasts.

5. Antihypertensive drugs and its relationship to inflammation

As discussed previously classicaly, the rennin-angiotensin system (RAS) has been considered a hormonal circulating system. The so-called systemic or circulating RAS plays a crucial role in the maintenance of blood pressure and electrolyte as well as fuid homeostasis15. This is mediated through its constrictive actions on vascular smooth muscle and by its influence on aldosterone secretion from the adrenal cortex, electrolyte transport in kidney, and on thirst as well as sodium appetite in the brain. In addition to its actions on the cardiovascular, renal, and nervous system, the expression of local RAS components in tissues such as the brain, kidneys, adrenals and gonads has led to the proposition that these components may either potentate systemic functions, or have entirely separate activities meeting the specific needs of these individual tissues.There is accumulating evidence that changes in tissue/organ-specific RAS may be associated with the pathophysiology of the respective tissue/organ functions (Ip et al., 2003).

The final goal of the RAS is the angiotensin II production that acts through the interaction with two pharmacologically defined receptor subtypes, namely type 1 (At1) and type 2 (At2) that are distributed in numerous target tissues and organs like pancreas, for example (Chan et al., 2000).

Some studies show that AT1 and AT2 receptors when activated by angiotensin II may lead to tissue that expresses inflammatory responses develop. This is the case of acute pancreatitis, which expresses the receptor AT1a more significantly than the receiver AT1b. In contrast, the AT2 receptor is most often responsible for these inflammatory responses more pronounced.

The role of RAS in the inflammatory process was further evidenced by the ability of an ACE inhibitor to suppress inflammation and subsequent tissue injury (Pupilli et al., 1999). Some studies suggest that losartan, an At1 blocker, and lisinopril, an angiotensin-converting enzyme (ACE) inhibitor, can inhibit both the liver fibrosis and portal hypertension occurring in secondary biliary cirrhosis by inhibiting hepatic stellate cells (HSCs) activation (Agarwal et al.,1993). Other studies in vitro of cultured pancreatic stellate cells have demonstrated that these cells exhibit morphological and functional features similar to cultured hepatic stellate cells, including positive SMA staining after a period of time in culture, increased proliferation in response to PDGF, and increased collagen synthesis in response to TGF-β (Gressner et al., 1995). So these stellate cells could trigger an inflammatory process in the tissue which is expressed.

Although other tissues, these stellate cells can not express the AT1 and AT2 receptors are widely distributed throughout the system and this can lead to a local inflammatory response by angiotensin II signaling. Given this relationship, it is necessary to comment briefly on the mechanism of action of antihypertensive agents shown below.

ACE Inhibitors: The essential effect of the agents belonging to this group of drugs is just the inhibition of the conversion of angiotensin I to II. In this respect ACE inhibitors are selective drugs, but because ACE has multiple substrates, these inhibitors may induce effects not related to reduced synthesis of angiotensin II. Among these various effects is the increased synthesis of bradykinin and prostaglandins that may contribute to the effects of ACE pharmacological inhibitors. A study by Silva, RB et al. (2010) in the Faculty of Medicine of Ribeirão Preto - FMRP / USP, Sao Paulo - Brazil, demonstrated that the application of drugs such as Lisinopril significantly reduced inflammatory response in an experimental model of acute pancreatitis, illustrating the relationship between the RAS and inflammation , figure 2.

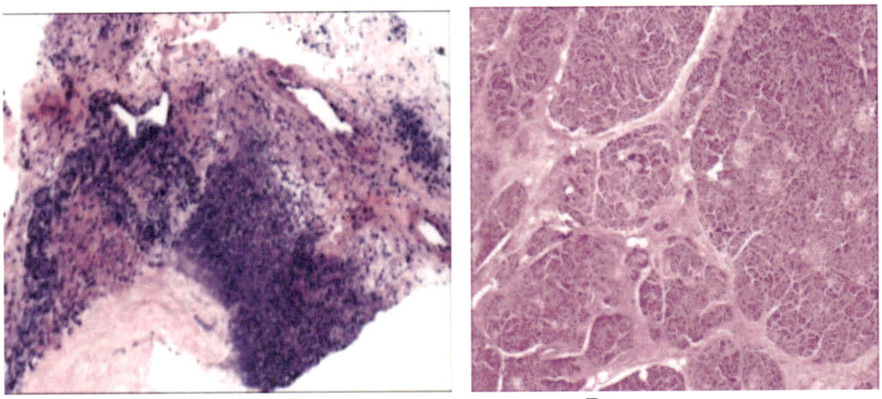

A B

Fig. 2. Map showing histopathological in (A) - The severe inflammatory process in the experimental group of acute pancreatitis and (B) - A significant reduction in inflammation in animals treated with lisinopril (Silva, R et al, 2010).

Captopril: Captopril was the first ACE inhibitor to be marketed. This drug has a bioavailability of about 75% and undergoes rapid absorption. Most of this drug is excreted in the urine, about 40 to 50% in the form of captopril and the remainder in the form of dimers. Captopril contains a sulfhydryl group.

Enalapril: enalapril is a pro-drug hydrolyzed by esterases in the liver. After this hydrolysis, enalapril is converted into a dicarboxylic acid which is known as enalaprilat a highly potent inhibitor of ACE.

Lisinopril: This drug differently than enalapril, it is active. In vitro studies show that Lisinopril is an ACE inhibitor slightly more potent than enalaprilat. Our study showed that this drug also has significant anti-inflammatory effects, but these results we have shown this relationship only in a specific experimental model of acute pancreatitis, requiring a slightly larger study, to ascertain whether this behavior also occurs in human beings. Lisinopril does not accumulate in the tissues.

Fosinopril: This drug contains a phosphinate group that binds to the active site of ACE. Liver esterase is cleaved and, with this prodrug that is converted to fosinopril, more potent than captopril and less potent than enalaprilat.

In pathological conditions such as hypertension, ACE inhibitors promote the reduction of systemic vascular resistance and various hypertensive states. This effect, as mentioned above arises from the action of reducing the production of angiotensin II, thereby reducing their pressor effects and vascular remodeling. But what must be understood is that angiotensin II has several other effects not only of increased blood pressure. These effects range from increased expression of proto-oncogene to the inflammation process. In the last decade studies have shown a strong relationship that RAS blockers possess anti atherosclerosis not only by regulating blood pressure, but also for its anti-inflammatory and antioxidant (Montecucco et al, 2009 and Schmieder et al, 2007). In this sense it is observed that studies that angiotensin II also acts on the expression of adhesion molecules such as intracellular adhesion molecule (ICAM), vasocelular adhesion molecule (VCAM), the P-selectin molecules expressed in the inflammatory process, and promote the expression of chemokines, growth factors and cytokines. Our study showed that angiotensin promotes the activation of certain stellate cells, which promote active since the deposition of collagen formation and fibrosis. So regardless of the mechanisms involved ACE inhibitors have broad clinical utility as antihypertensive agents, but also has a great potential for the therapy of other vascular disorders, and it is observed in experimental models.

Similarly antagonists of angiotensin II receptor act in lowering blood pressure, but unlike the effects of ACE inhibitors are not from inhibition of angiotensin II formation, but inhibition of its effects by antagonism of this peptide . This class of drugs bind to the AT1 receptor with high affinity and, in general, are around 10,000 times more selective for this receptor than for the AT2. The pharmacology of these antagonists is well described in the literature. Goldman and Gilman shows that studies in vitro and in vivo of these drugs block the majority of the biological effects of angiotensin II such as contraction of vascular smooth muscle, fast pressor responses, slow pressor responses, thirst, release of vasopressin, aldosterone secretion , release of catecholamines by the adrenal glands, increased noradrenergic neurotransmission, increased sympathetic tone, impaired renal function, cellular hypertrophy and hyperplasia, and inhibit the activation of pancreatic stellate cells, protecting from injuries such as acute pancreatitis, the latter effect was observed by Silva, RB. et al, 2010. Drugs that make up this group are: *candesartan, eprosartan, ibesartan, losartan, olmesartan, telmisartan and valsartan.*

Given this overview of the RAS and its relation to inflammation, we can observe that the drugs used to treat hypertension are consistent with the possible protective effects of a serial of inflammatory disorders. However the application of these to treat acute problems like apancreatite, for example, is not observed, but promising results from several studies, show that these drugs may be important in the treatment of various inflammatory disorders, is atherosclerosis, ischemia , or even pancreatitis. We observed in our work that pancreatic stellate cells respond to the action of angiotensin II (Figure 3 and 4) and in addition, we observed that these respond directly, because these cells have receptors for angiotensin II AT1 as illustrating the existence of even a Local RAS, regulating the vasculature of the tissue in question. Because of this, these drugs as mentioned above, could be a viable alternative to treat these other disorders.

In our study we observed that the strength pancreatic stellate cells in collagen production are involved during acute pancreatitis and possibly that these can become active cells through the action of angiotensin II produced by rennin-angiotensin system. However it has been suggested an increasingly close relationship between the RAS and the inflammatory process in this sense these studies indicate a relationship of therapy used to treat hypertension is also feasible in other disorders such as inflammatory problems.

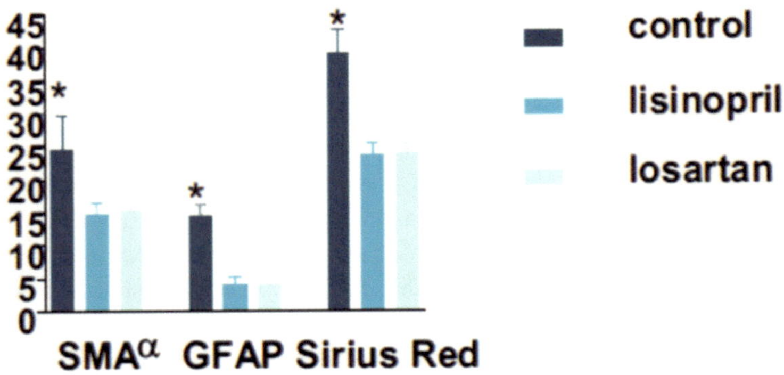

Fig. 3. Comparison of the number of pancreatic stellate cells marked for alpha-smooth muscle actin (α-SMA) and fibrillary acidic protein glial (GFAP), and the percentage of points scored by used. The (PS), between the pancreas of control rats treated with lisinopril and losartan. The bars represent the mean ± SD. * P <0.001, compared to the treaties.

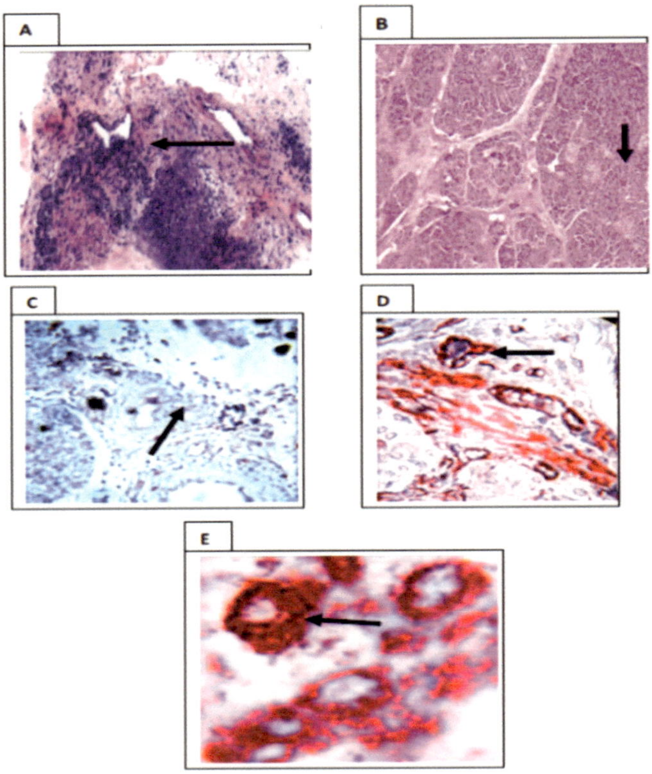

Fig. 4. Slides stained by hematoxylin and eosin (A) to inflammatory analysis have showed more neutrophylic inflammatory infiltrate in sample of control group measured in [purple]. Moreover slides stained by Sirius red (B) have showed more collagen deposit in the animals of control group too showed in [eosinofilic]. In the group treated (C) and stained by immunohistochemical staining method (GFAP or α-SMA) have less PSCs activated marked in [blue] compared with animals control (D and E) which have more PSCs activated measured in [red] ($p<0.05$)

6. References

Agarwal N, Pitchumoni CS. Acute pancreatitis: a multisystem disease. Gastrenterologist. 1993;1:115-28

Bachem MG, Schneider E, Groß H, Weidenbach H, Schmid RM, Menke A, Siech M, Beger H, Grünert A, Adler G. Identification, culture, and characterisation of pancreatic stellate cells in rats and humans. *Gastroenterology* 1998, 115:421-432.

Barros,R., Ramalho, FS e Ramalho, LN. The effect of anti-hypertensive drugs on the obstructive pancreatitis in rats. *Acta Cirurgica Brasileira* 2010, 25:396 - 400

Beierwaltes WH. The role of calcium in the regulation of renin secretion. *Am J Physiol Renal Physiol* 2009, 1-36.

Chan WP, Fung ML, Nobiling R, Leung PS. Activation of local rennin- angiotensin system by chronic hypoxia. Molec Cell Endocrinol. 2000;160:107-14

Chappell MC, Millsted A, Diz DI, Brosnihan KB, Ferrario CM: Evidence for an intrinsic angiotensin system in the canine pancreas. *J Hypertens* 1991, 9:751-759.

De Gasparo M, Catt KJ, Inagami T, Wright JW, Unger TH. The angiotensin II receptors. *Pharmacol Rev.* 2000;52:415-72.

Donoghue,M., Hsieh,F., Baronas, E., *et al.* A novel angiotensin –converting enzyme related carboxypeptidase (ACE2) convert angiotensin 1 to angiotensin (1-9). Circ. Res., 2000, 87:E1-E9.

Goldman and Gilman. The Pharmacological Basis Therapeutics. The Ed. MacGraw - Hill Companies, 11ªedition. 2007

Graninger M., Reiter R., Drucker C., Minar E., Jilma B. "Angiotensin receptor blockade decreasesmarkers of vascular inflammation," Journal of Cardiovascular Pharmacology 2004, 44:335–339.

Hackenthal E, Paul M, Ganten D, Taugner R. Morphology, physiology, and molecular biology of rennin secretion. *Physiol Rev.* 1990;4:1067-116.

Hama K, Ohnishi H, Yasuda H, Ueda N, Mashima H, Satoh Y, Hanat-suka K, Kita H, Ohashi A, Tamada K, Sugano K. Angiotensin II stimulates DNA synthesis of rat pancreatic stellate cells by activating ERK through EGF receptor transactivation. Bio-chem Biophys Res. Commun 2004, 315:905-911.

Ip SP, Kwan PC, Williams CH, Pang S, Hooper NM, Leung PS. Changes of angiotensin - converting enzyme activity in the pancreas of chronic hypoxia and acute pancreatitis. Int J Biochem Cell Biol. 2003;35:944-54.

Jacoby D.S. and Rader D.J. "Renin-angiotensin system and atherothrombotic disease: from genes to treatment," Archives of Internal Medicine, vol. 163, no. 10, pp. 1155–1164, 2003.

Leung PS, Chan HC & Wong PYD. Immunohistochemical localization of angiotensin II in the mouse pancreas. Histochemical Journal 1998, 30: 21–25.

Leung PS, Chan WP, Wong TP, Sernia C Expression and localization of renin–angiotensin system in the rat pancreas. Journal of Endocrinology 1999, 160:13–19.

Leung PS, Carlsson PO. Tissue renin–angiotensin system: its expression, localization, regulation and potential role in the pancreas. J Mol Endocrinol 2000, 166:121–8.

Montecucco F., Pende A., Mach F. The Renin-Angiotensin SystemModulates Inflammatory Processes in Atherosclerosis: Evidence from Basic Research and Clinical Studies. Mediators of Inflammation, 2009, 1-13.

Pupilli C, Lasagni L, Romagnani P, Bellini F, Mannelli M, Misciglia N, Mavilia C, Vellei U, Villari D, Serio M. Angiotensin II stimulates the synthesis and secretion of vascular permeability factor/vascular endothelial growth factor in human mesangial cells. J Am Soc Nephrol. 1999;10:245-55

Williams B, Baker AQ, Gallacher B, Lodwick D. Angiotensin II increases vascular permeability factor gene expression by human vascular smooth muscle cells. *Hypertension*. 1995;5:913-7.

6

Pharmacokinetic Interactions of Antihypertensive Drugs with Citrus Juices

Yoshihiro Uesawa
Meiji Pharmaceutical University, Japan

1. Introduction

It has been known that citrus juices cause pharmaceutical interactions with various kinds of medications. The citrus juice interactions are broadly divided into 2 types which are with increasing and decreasing of drug concentrations in plasma. That is, both types are categorized into pharmacokinetic interactions. In the "increasing" type interactions, grapefruit juice is the most important in the juices. Grapefruit juice makes an increase in the plasma drug concentrations due to the suppression of intestinal metabolization of the drugs. Since the danger of concomitant administration of drugs and grapefruit juice was discovered in 1989, drinking of the juice has been controlled in patients undergoing pharmaceutical therapies. The targeted medications for the restriction ranges from antilipemics to immunosuppressants. Antihypertensive drugs are one of the typical categories of drugs affected by such interaction. A feature of said drugs is that they are characterized as substrates of Cytochrome P-450 3A, the most important-drug metabolizing enzyme in the intestines. Dihydropyridine calcium channel antagonists, as well as verapamil in the antihypertensive drugs was representative of drug categories with such property. In this chapter, grapefruit juice interactions were described, and the latest knowledge presented, as a results of research utilizing statistical investigations with dihydropyridines. On the other hand, information about the "decreasing" type of interactions has been reported in a limited number of research results. Some clinical studies related to β-adrenergic-blocking agents (antihypertensives) such as celiprolol as well as fexofenadine (antihistamine), it was discovered that citrus juices such as orange juice and grapefruit juice reduce intestinal absorption of the drugs. In this chapter, results of the studies of the interactions are explained; and the research attributing an important ingredient in orange juice in the interaction with the β-blocker, is described.

2. Grapefruit juice interactions related to the increase of plasma drug concentrations

In 1989, Bailey and colleagues used grapefruit juice (GFJ) to mask the taste of alcohol in a clinical trial of the interaction between alcohol and drugs. They found that plasma felodipine levels were higher in subjects given GFJ (Bailey, 1989); and in 1991, they published a similar work on both felodipine and nifedipine (Bailey, 1991). At present, GFJ must be avoided in patients receiving certain drugs to prevent this interaction (Figure 1).

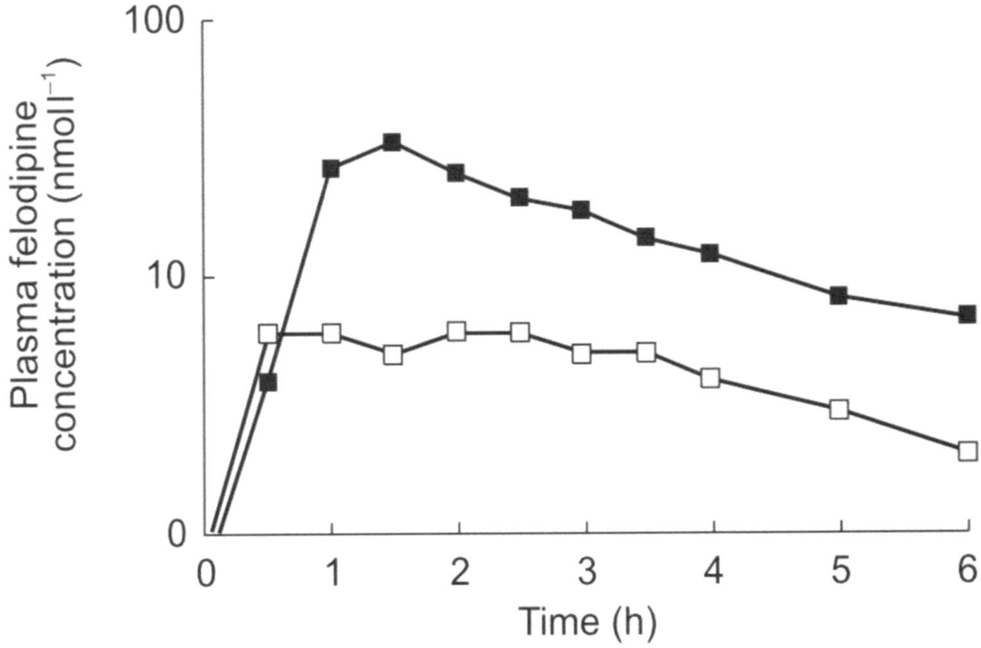

Felodipine 5 mg tablet was administered with 350 mL double-strength GFJ (black squares) or water (white squares). This figure was cited from the literature (Bailey, 1998)

Fig. 1. Plasma felodipine concentration-time profile.

2.1 Antihypertensive drugs related with the GFJ- interactions

Concomitant administration of GFJ with a variety of drugs including antihypertensive drugs results in enhancement of plasma concentrations of the drugs. The first example of a GFJ interaction was an increase in levels of the dihydropyridine calcium channel antagonists, felodipine and nifedipine (Bailey et al., 1991), but at least 13 drugs in this category also interact with GFJ: amlodipine (Josefsson, 1996), azelnidipine (Hirashima, 2006), benidipine (Ohnishi, 2006), cilnidipine (Ohnishi et al., 2006), efonidipine (Yajima, 2003), felodipine (Bailey et al., 1991), manidipine (Sugawara, 1996), nicardipine (Uno, 2000), nifedipine (Bailey et al., 1991), nimodipine (Fuhr, 1998), nisoldipine (Bailey, 1993b), nitrendipine (Soons, 1991), and pranidipine (Hashimoto, 1998). GFJ can interact with other diverse medicines such as verapamil (Ho, 2000) (calcium channel antagonist), simvastatin (Lilja, 1998) (HMG-CoA reductase inhibitor), and losartan (Zaidenstein, 2001) (angiotensin II receptor blocker).

2.2 The mechanism of GFJ-drug interactions

Most interacting drugs are substrates of Cytochrome P-450 3A (CYP3A). CYP3A is an important drug oxidation enzyme in human liver and the small intestine, and metabolizes 50% of commercially available drugs. CYP3A blocks the intestinal absorption of small-molecule xenobiotics from drugs and food and drink components. GFJ is a suicidal substrate of this enzyme (Lown, 1997; Schmiedlin-Ren, 1997). A single glassful of GFJ can decrease CYP3A activity by 47% (Lown et al., 1997), drastically increasing the fractional absorption of CYP3A substrates depending on other drug properties.

2.3 GFJ components involved in drug interactions

2.3.1 Construction of the estimation model on the CYP3A inhibitory effect of GFJ

When first discovered, naringin (NG), a high concentration ingredient in GFJ (Kane & Lipsky, 2000), and naringenin, an aglycone of naringin, were considered as the candidates that are most responsible for the interactions (Guengerich & Kim, 1990; Fuhr, 1993). The discovery of these components indicated CYP3A inhibition in *in vitro* experiments (Guengerich & Kim, 1990). However, studies on treatments with drugs combined with NG revealed that it does not contribute to the interactions (Bailey, 1993a). Currently, furanocoumarin derivatives such as bergamottin (BG) (He, 1998; Eagling, 1999; Malhotra, 2001; Mohri & Uesawa, 2001a; Goosen, 2004; Paine, 2004; Girennavar, 2006), 6′,7′-dihydroxybergamottin (DHB) (Eagling et al., 1999; Malhotra et al., 2001; Paine et al., 2004; Girennavar et al., 2006), and paradisins (Tassaneeyakul, 2000; Girennavar et al., 2006) are putative ingredients implicated in the interactions. The enzymatic inhibitory effects of these ingredients have been studied. However, the contributing rate of each derivative in the pharmaceutical interaction or CYP3A inhibitory effect was still being debated.

Estimation of the amount of contribution to the inhibitory effect by the purified ingredients might be difficult because concentrations of the furanocoumarins in GFJ vary with the brand of juice (Uesawa, 2008; Uesawa & Mohri, 2008b). While it is considered that estimation of the interaction potential on each GFJ brand is useful to select drinkable brands for patients undergoing pharmaceutical treatment, the complexity of interactive mechanisms with plural causative ingredients makes such estimation difficult. Therefore, we investigated the relationships between CYP3A inhibitory effects in a variety of GFJs and the concentrations of the ingredients, to construct a prediction model for the interaction potentials of GFJ (Uesawa, 2011a). Concentrations of bergaptol (BT), BG, DHB, NG, and naringenin in 23 kinds of GFJ were determined with high-performance liquid chromatography (HPLC) systems, equipped with photodiode array and electrospray ionization mass spectrometric detectors. Furthermore, inhibitory effects on CYP3A activity were measured based on the initial rate for testosterone 6β-hydroxylation in the presence of each GFJ. The concentrations of bergaptol, DHB, BG, NG, and naringenin in GFJ used in this study were 31.6, 4.97, 10.4, 364, and 1.37 μM, respectively. Addition of the juice to the reaction mixtures reduced human CYP3A activities to 32.7 % of the control. The residual activities underwent a multitude of changes, depending on the GFJ sample. The relationship between the concentration of 5 kinds of ingredients present in GFJ and their residual activities on CYP3A were studied to investigate the cause of the variability.

Figure 2 shows stacker plots between bergaptol, DHB, BG, NG, and naringenin concentrations, and the remaining CYP3A activities in the 23 kinds of GFJ. All the ingredients except bergaptol showed significant negative relationships for the residual activities. Multiple linear regression analysis was performed to estimate the contribution ratios of the GFJ-ingredients to the inhibitory effects on CYP3A activity. A multiple regression model where concentrations of DHB, BG, and NG were used as the significant variables was constructed (Figure 3). The inhibitory effects of GFJ on CYP3A activities could be attributed to almost all these ingredients because the contribution ratio in the above equation was 88% (Figure 3). Standardized partial regression coefficients of DHB, BG, and NG suggest that the order of contribution of the ingredients in the whole juice to the CYP3A inhibition is in the order of DHB>BG>>NG. We believe that the furanocoumarins including DHB and BG were important factors in the GFJ interactions, compared with the other components such as flavonoid. Our findings suggest that quantitative determination of DHB and BG was a useful method for brief assessment of GFJ brands in pharmaceutical interactions.

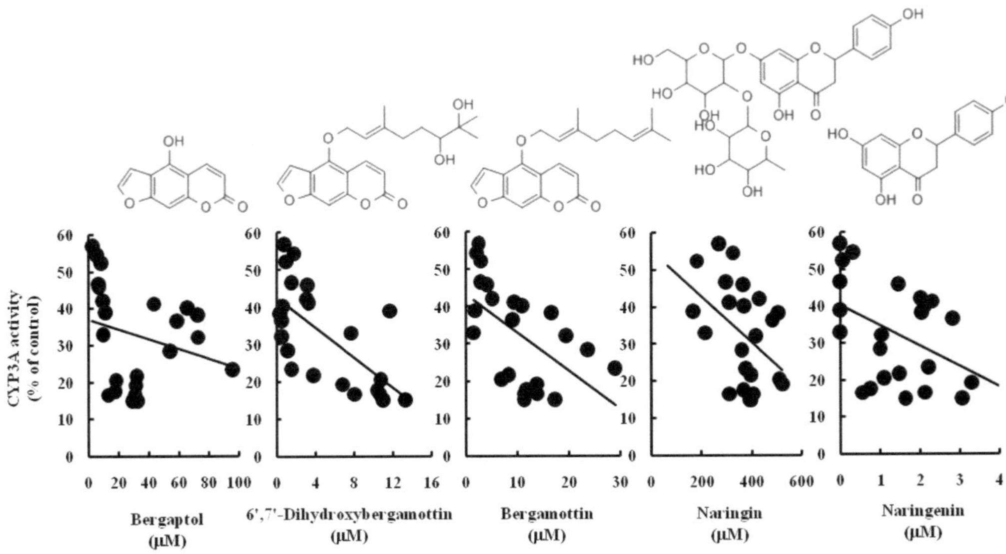

This figure was cited from the literature (Uesawa et al., 2011a).

Fig. 2. Plots of concentrations of ingredients vs. observed CYP3A activities (% of control) with 23 kinds of GFJ.

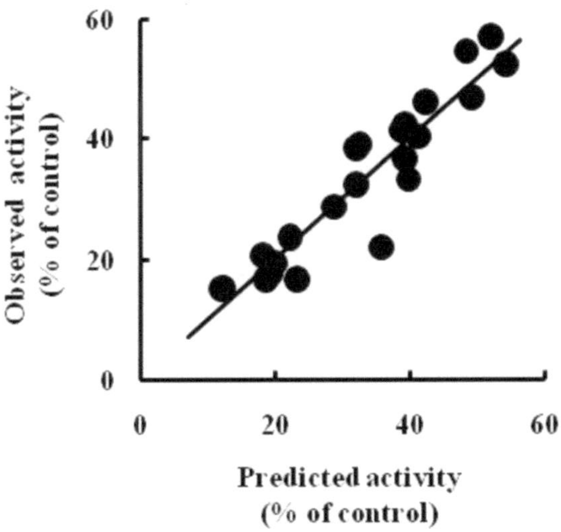

Activity = 65.5 - 2.18DHB - 0.936BG - 0.0338NG (R^2 = 0.875)
In the equation, "activity" indicates the remaining CYP3A activity in the reaction mixture added to each GFJ. "DHB", "BG", and "NG" indicate the respective concentrations (μM) in each GFJ.
This figure was cited from the literature (Uesawa et al., 2011a).

Fig. 3. Multiple linear regression between predicted and observed CYP3A activities (% of control) with 23 kinds of GFJ.

2.3.2 QSAR analysis of the inhibitory effects of furanocoumarin derivatives on CYP3A activities

Furanocoumarin derivatives (FCs) exist in citrus fruits such as lime (Saita, 2004) and pomelo (Uesawa & Mohri, 2005) and umbellifers (Fujioka, 1999) as well as grapefruit. Like grapefruit, foods, drinks, and medicines from these plants might affect drug absorption. In fact, it was reported that pomelo juice, which has 8 kinds of FCs (Uesawa & Mohri, 2005), increased the bioavailability of cyclosporine A (Grenier, 2006). In one article, IC_{50} values of a variety of FCs on testosterone-6-ß hydroxylation were evaluated using human liver microsomes as the inhibitory effects (Guo, 2000). However, some points were still unclear regarding the relationship between the CYP-inhibitory effects and physicochemical profiles of FCs. Therefore, the quantitative structure-activity relationship (QSAR) study on the CYP3A inhibitory effects of FCs was designed such that the structural, physicochemical, and quantum chemical properties on FCs can be elucidated by use of computational chemical predictions (Uesawa & Mohri, 2010). Common logarithmic IC_{50} values of human liver microsomal testosterone 6-ß-hydroxylations were configured as objective variables. A variety of structural, physicochemical, and quantum chemical descriptors were computed from 2D and optimized 3D structures in the 37 FCs (Figure 4) as explanatory variables. Simple and multiple linear regression analyses were used to evaluate these parameters. IC_{50} values were taken from the literature and used as parameters that indicate the CYP3A inhibitory effect of the 37 kinds of FCs (Guo et al., 2000). Common logarithms of the parameters (log IC_{50}) were utilized as objective variables in the present regression analyses.

We attempted to construct multiple regression equations using descriptors and their square values that were calculated in this study. As a result, the best model was a quadratic function with log P and log P^2 (Figure 5).

The final model is

$$\text{Log } IC_{50}=1.44-0.385\text{AlogP}+0.0528(\text{AlogP}-4.00)^2$$

Variation of log IC_{50} values was interpretable in log P because the contribution ratio of the regression model constructed from log P was 81.2% for 36 FCs except FC24 (bergamottin). The presence of an outlier on bergamottin suggests that unknown physicochemical properties might differentiate the inhibitory effects of bergamottin from that of the other FCs. The structural characteristics of bergamottin are difficult to distinguish from those of the other FCs such as FC25, FC26, and FC27 with log P values close to that of bergamottin. On the other hand, we have reported that an effect of bergamottin on nifedipine oxidation activity with rat-liver microsomes was greater than those of FC26 (6′,7′-dihydroxybergamottin), FC2 (bergapten), and bergaptol (Mohri & Uesawa, 2001a). Herein, logP values of 6′,7′-dihydroxybergamottin, bergapten and bergaptol, 3.41, 2.19 and 1.94, respectively, were lower than bergamottin's 5.48. This order of inhibitory effects of the FCs also perfectly correlates with the order from the model equation. In the model, the IC_{50} value of bergamottin was estimated at 280nM. In fact, it became evident that bergamottin is one component involved in the GFJ-drug interaction that results in inhibition of the CYP3A enzyme in the intestinal lumen *in vivo* (Goosen et al., 2004). Goosen et al. reported significant increase in felodipine AUC, area under the plasma concentration-time curve, when subjects co-administered bergamottin at the same concentration of GFJ. These findings and our estimation from the regression model suggest that bergamottin could be an important factor in GFJ-interactions.

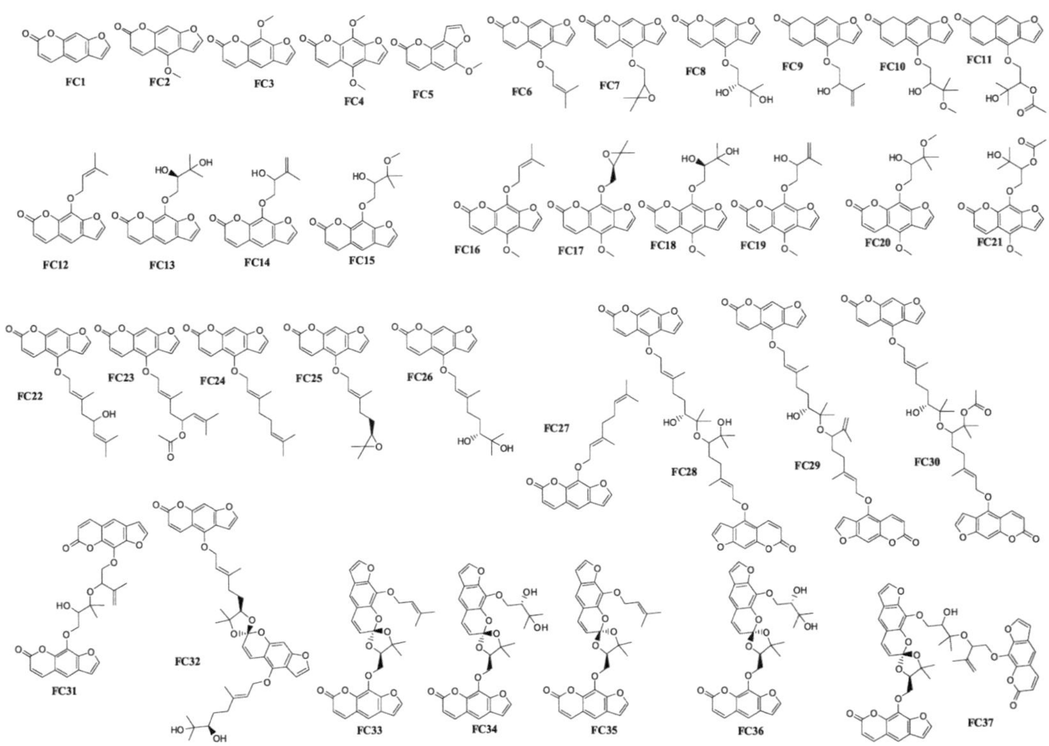

Fig. 4. Chemical structures of FCs.

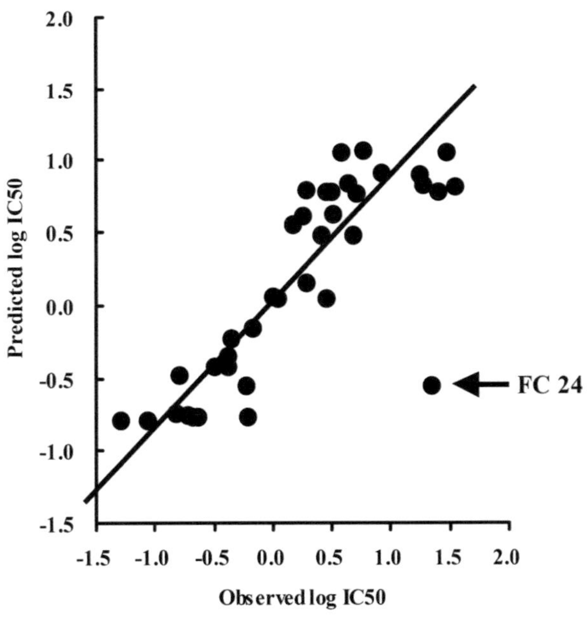

This figure was cited from the literature (Uesawa & Mohri, 2010)

Fig. 5. Linear regression between predicted and observed values of IC_{50} in CYP3A activities of FCs obtained in the model with AlogP and $AlogP^2$.

2.4 Meta-analyses of studies of GFJ interactions with dihydropyridine drugs

Studies on GFJ interaction are known to vary widely. We believed that studies with such a wide deviation should be integrated (Uesawa, 2011b). Amlodipine, efonidipine, manidipine, felodipine, nifedipine, and nisoldipine were mentioned in 2 reports (Josefsson et al., 1996; Vincent, 2000), 3 reports (Mimura, 1998, 2000; Yajima et al., 2003), 2 reports (Sugawara, 1996; Uno, 2006), 12 reports (Bailey et al., 1991, 1993a, 1998; Edgar, 1992; Bailey, 1995, 1996, 2000, 2003; Lundahl, 1995, 1997; Lown et al., 1997; Goosen et al., 2004), 6 reports (Bailey et al., 1991, 1993a; Rashid, 1993, 1995; Sigusch, 1994; Azuma, 1996; Ohtani, 2002), and 4 reports (Bailey et al., 1993a, b; Azuma et al., 1996; Takanaga, 2000; Ohtani et al., 2002), respectively (Table 1). Therefore, the GFJ interaction of each drug in these reports was set up as a target of the meta-analysis. In most of the reports on all drugs analyzed in this study, concomitant administration of GFJ resulted in the increment of concentrations and AUCs on the drugs in plasma compared with that of the control groups. There are some reports without significant increase in AUC for 3 kinds of dihydropyridine drugs, namely, efonidipine, nifedipine, and amlodipine with concomitant intake of GFJ (Figure 7, 8, and 12). There were significant increases in AUCs in the groups that administered GFJ compared with those that administered water for efonidipine, felodipine, nifedipine, manidipine, and nisoldipine (Figure 7-11). On the other hand, a meta-analysis of amlodipine showed no significant interaction (Figure 12). All other single studies on azelnidipine, benidipine, cilnidipine, nicardipine, nimodipine, nitrendipine, and pranidipine showed significant increases in AUCs in the groups that administered GFJ, compared with the control groups. Amlodipine was considered the only safe medication among all the dihydropyridine drugs reported to date. The numbers of studies for manidipine, amlodipine and efonidipine are 2, 2, and 3, respectively. The quality of the results of meta-analyses based on these dihydropyridines might not be sufficient. Progress of additional studies is expected.

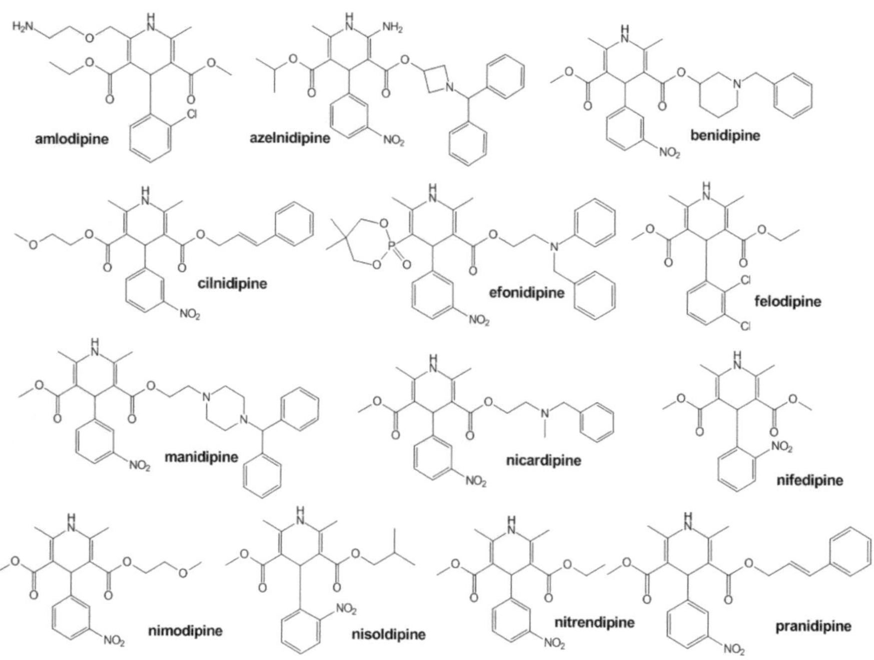

Fig. 6. Chemical structures of dihydropyridines.

Drug	Author	Publication year	Jadad	GFJ-administration n	Dose (mg)	GFJ (mL)	AUC (nmol x h/L/mg)	mean AUC	Control n	Dose (mg)	AUC (nmol x h/L/mg)	mean AUC	mean AUC ratio
amlodipine	Josefsson	1996	3	12	5	250	70.44 ± 18.59	74.56	12	5	61.63 ± 14.67	67.90	1.10
amlodipine	Vincent	2000	3	20	10	240	77.04 ± 18.59		20	10	71.66 ± 14.19		
azelnidipine	Hirashima	2006	2	8	8	250	31.73 ± 9.41	31.73	8	8	9.68 ± 2.01	9.68	3.28
benidipine	Coniel	1995	0	6	4	200	1.57	1.57	6	4	0.98	0.98	1.59
cilnidipine	Watanabe	1999	0	6	10	200	25.69	25.69	6	10	11.31	11.31	2.27
efonidipine	Mimura	1998	1	5	20	200	3.42 ± 1.16	3.81	5	20	2.01 ± 0.92	2.27	1.68
efonidipine	Mimura	2000	1	4	20	250	1.31 ± 0.65		5	20	1.09 ± 0.83		
efonidipine	Yajima	2003	2	19	40	250	4.44 ± 1.73		19	40	2.65 ± 1.12		
felodipine	Bailey	1991	3	6	5	500	20.60 ± 7.35	11.20	6	5	8.20 ± 3.92	5.76	1.94
felodipine	Edgar	1992	3	9	5	200	13.00 ± 5.26		9	5	4.56 ± 2.12		
felodipine	Bailey	1993	3	9	5	200	8.20 ± 3.60		9	5	4.40 ± 2.40		
felodipine	Bailey	1995	3	12	10	250	14.73 ± 5.70		12	10	7.31 ± 2.99		
felodipine	Lundahl	1995	3	9	10	200	14.59 ± 3.03		9	10	10.17 ± 2.12		
felodipine	Bailey	1996	3	12	10	250	12.93 ± 3.79		12	10	6.71 ± 3.07		
felodipine	Lown	1997	1	10	10	237	7.64 ± 1.56		10	10	3.53 ± 2.16		
felodipine	Lundahl	1997	3	12	10	150	11.50 ± 3.53		12	10	6.68 ± 2.08		
felodipine	Bailey	1998	3	12	10	250	13.00 ± 5.20		12	10	5.30 ± 2.42		
felodipine	Bailey	2000	3	12	10	250	5.40 ± 2.77		12	10	2.50 ± 1.73		
felodipine	Bailey	2003	2	8	10	250	6.50 ± 3.11		8	10	3.60 ± 2.26		
felodipine	Goosen	2004	3	11	5	250	9.20 ± 2.56		11	5	6.82 ± 2.04		
manidipine	Sugawara	1996	0	6	40		2.92 ± 1.16	3.35	6	40	1.24 ± 0.21	1.33	2.51
manidipine	Uno	2006	2	7	40	250	3.71 ± 1.20		7	40	1.42 ± 0.30		
nicardipine	Uno	2000	2	6	40	300	21.04 ± 7.40	21.04	6	40	13.47 ± 2.58	13.47	1.56
nifedipine	Bailey	1991	3	6	10	500	62.70 ± 37.23	76.13	6	10	46.40 ± 22.54	57.54	1.32
nifedipine	Rashid	1993	3	8	10	400	92.40 ± 48.96		8	10	62.95 ± 30.00		
nifedipine	Sigusch	1994	3	10	20	200	47.35 ± 20.79		10	20	23.39 ± 12.13		
nifedipine	Rashid	1995	3	8	10	400	86.91 ± 27.43		8	10	55.15 ± 17.04		
nifedipine	Azuma	1996	3	8	20	250	101.12 ± 64.72		8	20	109.78 ± 104.77		
nifedipine	Ohtani	2002	1	8	20	227	70.14 ± 19.13		8	20	53.35 ± 12.04		
nimodipine	Fuhr	1998	2	8	30	250	117.78 ± 1.92	117.78	8	30	77.84 ± 1.61	77.84	1.51
nisoldipine	Bailey	1993	3	12	20	250	4.51 ± 2.50	5.48	12	20	2.56 ± 0.94	2.24	2.45
nisoldipine	Azuma	1996	3	8	10	250	6.59 ± 2.19		8	10	1.85 ± 1.74		
nisoldipine	Takanaga	2000	1	8	5	200	8.26 ± 3.35		8	10	2.01 ± 0.80		
nisoldipine	Ohtani	2002	1	8	10	227	3.05 ± 0.79		8	10	2.37 ± 0.97		
nitrendipine	Soon	1991	3	9	20	150	9.95 ± 8.77	9.95	9	20	4.41 ± 2.75	4.41	2.25
Pranidipine	Hashimoto	1998	1	8	2	250	39.70 ± 17.43	39.70	8	2	23.59 ± 13.29	23.59	1.68

Volume of double strength GFJ was converted to that of single strength GFJ. The method for calculating mean AUC is described in Methods. This table was cited from the literature (Uesawa et al., 2011b).

Table 1. Reported Pharmacokinetic Interactions of Dihydropyridines Following Consumption of GFJ in humans.

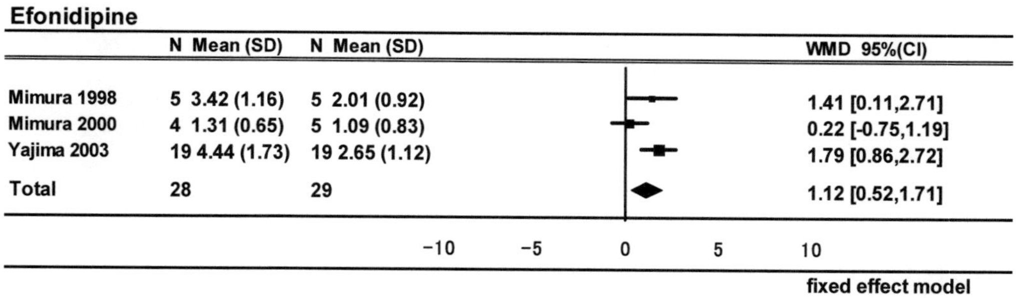

WMD and the 95% CI were calculated by the general variance-based method. This figure was cited from the literature (Uesawa et al., 2011b).

Fig. 7. Forest plot of the average difference of efonidipine AUC (nmol · h/L/mg dose) and the corresponding 95% CI from the studies included in the meta-analysis of GFJ-interactions.

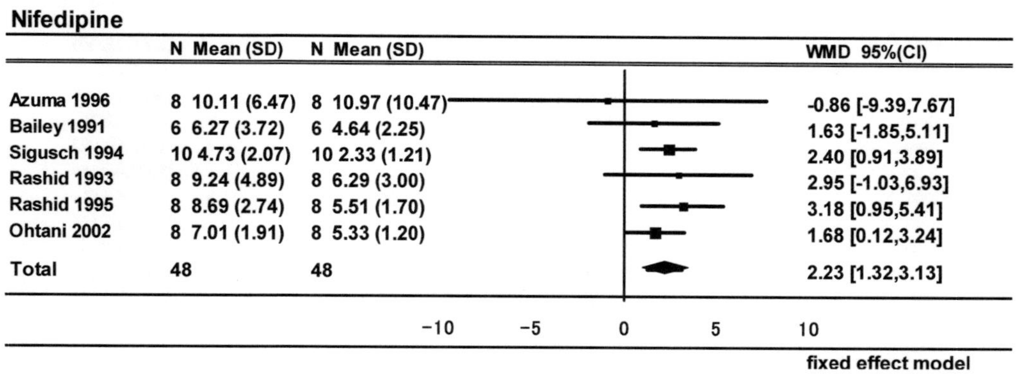

WMD and the 95% CI were calculated by the general variance-based method. This figure was cited from the literature (Uesawa et al., 2011b).

Fig. 8. Forest plot of the average difference of nifedipine AUC (nmol · h/L/mg dose) and the corresponding 95% CI from the studies included in the meta-analysis of GFJ-interactions.

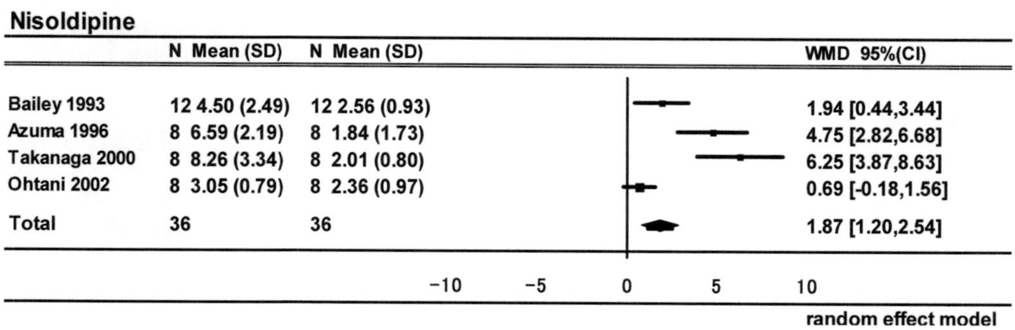

WMD and the 95% CI were calculated by the general variance-based method. This figure was cited from the literature (Uesawa et al., 2011b).

Fig. 9. Forest plot of the average difference of nisoldipine AUC (nmol · h/L/mg dose) and the corresponding 95% CI from the studies included in the meta-analysis of GFJ-interactions.

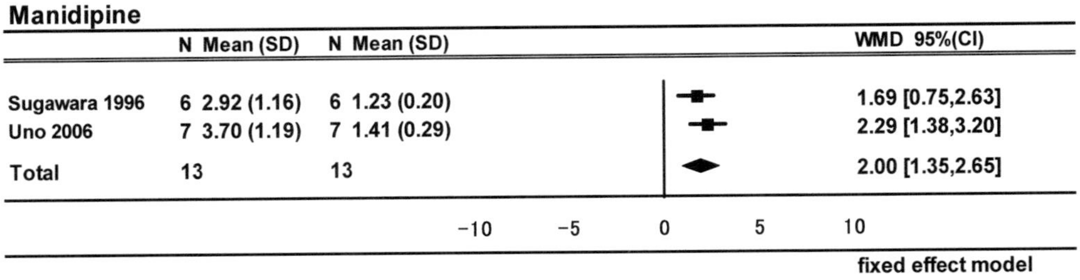

WMD and the 95% CI were calculated by the general variance-based method. This figure was cited from the literature (Uesawa et al., 2011b).

Fig. 10. Forest plot of the average difference of manidipine AUC (nmol · h/L/mg dose) and the corresponding 95% CI from the studies included in the meta-analysis of GFJ-interactions.

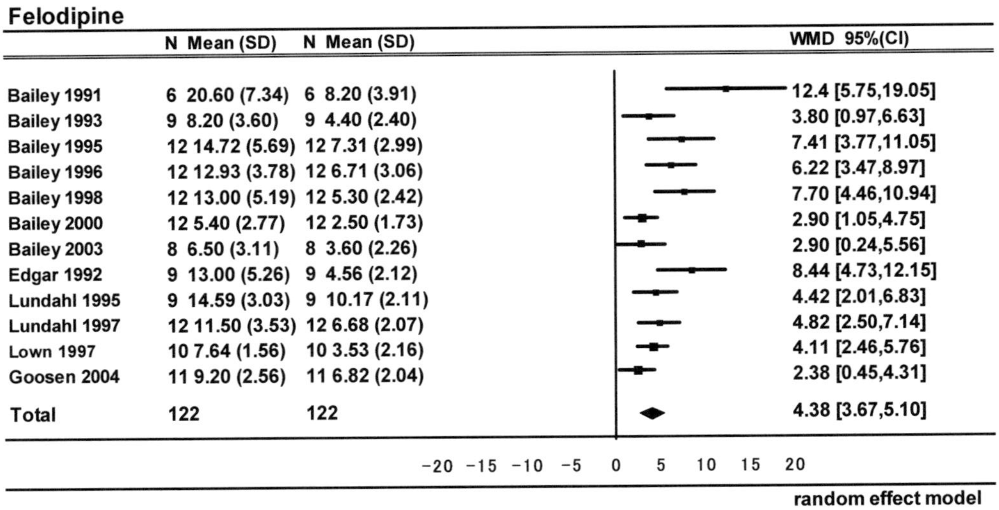

WMD and the 95% CI were calculated by the general variance-based method. This figure was cited from the literature (Uesawa et al., 2011b).

Fig. 11. Forest plot of the average difference of felodipine AUC (nmol · h/L/mg dose) and the corresponding 95% CI from the studies included in the meta-analysis of GFJ-interactions.

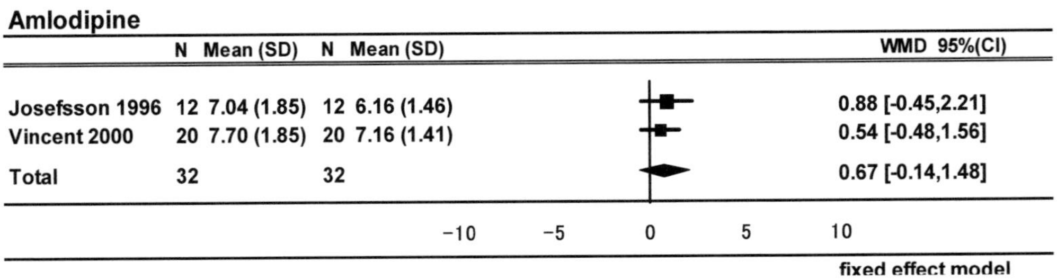

WMD and the 95% CI were calculated by the general variance-based method. This figure was cited from the literature (Uesawa et al., 2011b).

Fig. 12. Forest plot of the average difference of amlodipine AUC (nmol · h/L/mg dose) and the corresponding 95% CI from the studies included in the meta-analysis of GFJ-interactions.

2.5 Relationship between lipophilicities of 1,4-dihydropyridine derivatives and pharmacokinetic interaction strengths with GFJ

The structural and physicochemical properties of currently used 1,4-Dihydropyridine calcium channel antagonists vary significantly. However, little was known about the correlation between the structures and the clinical interaction strengths (CISs). Therefore analysis was performed using the predictive properties calculated from the chemical structures and the reported pharmacokinetic interactions with GFJ consumption (Uesawa & Mohri, 2008c). Thirteen dihydropyridines - amlodipine, azelnidipine, benidipine, cilnidipine, efonidipine, felodipine, manidipine, nicardipine, nifedipine, nimodipine, nisoldipine, nitrendipine, and pranidipine - on which there were confirmable reports of pharmacokinetic interactions with GFJ, were selected for analysis. CISs were defined as common logarithmic values of the AUC increasing ratio, in which the AUC of each dihydropyridine with GFJ consumption was divided by the corresponding control AUC. The first report with a significant interaction with GFJ intake for each drug was referred to the AUC value to avoid the variation of CIS in publication bias. Three types of predicted logP values, ALOGPs (Tetko & Tanchuk, 2002), ClogP (Chou & Jurs, 1979), and XLOGP (Wang, 1997), and seven other physicochemical properties, water diffusion, molecular volume, molecular polarization, molecular density, refractive index, topologic polar surface area, and calculated molar refractivity, were calculated from the chemical structures. Analyses using the linear least-squares method for relationship between the physicochemical properties and CISs represent each logP value, CLogP, ALOGPs, and XLOGP, but not water diffusion, molecular volume, molecular polarization, molecular density, refractive index, topologic polar surface area, and calculated molar refractivity, correlated with CIS:

$$CIS = 0.0822ALOGPs - 0.0651,\ r = 0.626;\ CIS = 0.0569ClogP - 0.0276,\ r = 0.592;\ CIS = 0.0582XLOGP + 0.0272,\ r = 0.587 \text{ (Figure 13)}$$

Dihydropyridines have a 1,4-dihydropyridine ring as a common structure. This partial structure is characterized by substrates of cytochrome P-450, which form a pyridine ring as a result of the enzymatic reaction (Baarnhielm, 1984; Rush, 1986; Terashita, 1987). The aromatic-ring formation reaction is caused by the dihydropyridines losing their calcium antagonistic effect. Dihydropyridines used in clinical practice have a variety of chemical structures, suggesting various physicochemical and pharmacokinetic properties. In this study, findings from clinical trials were used in calculating CISs, and the conditions of pharmacokinetic investigation in the reports differed, resulting in errors among pharmacokinetic data. Nevertheless, the results showed that the relationship between CISs and the predicted logP values for the 13 dihydropyridines indicated significant correlation, which was expressed as simple linear regression formulae. These results suggest that the lipophilicity of the drugs is an important factor in the interactions.

It is considered that the clearance of dihydropyridines in first-pass metabolism is regulated by intestinal and hepatic intrinsic clearance. Because the target organ of GFJ is the intestine, it has been speculated that dihydropyridine with a higher contribution ratio of intestinal clearance in the first pass has stronger interaction with the concomitant consumption of GFJ. Ohnishi *et al.* reported that the plasma protein-binding ratio correlated with an increasing ratio of AUC for calcium-blocking agents with the consumption of GFJ (Ohnishi et al., 2006). This suggested the possibility that drugs that have higher plasma unbound fractions reflect a higher percentage of contribution of the intestinal metabolism in first-pass effect due to a lower hepatic extraction ratio. LogP values are a parameter-informed correlation with the plasma protein binding of drugs (Kiehs, 1966; Yamazaki & Kanaoka, 2004) and, because of this, it is conceivable that the present results support the report showing a correlation between the extent of the interactions and protein-binding ratios. Furthermore, it is known that lipophilicity is one of the parameters contributing to absorption (Houston, 1975), distribution (Watanabe & Kozaki, 1978; Yamada, 1993), metabolism (Kim, 1991), and excretion (Cantelli-Forti, 1986; Yamada et al., 1993) in pharmacokinetics. For example, enzymatic affinities and kinetic properties in CYP oxidation of various compounds are regulated by the logP values of the substrates (Lewis, 2000). Therefore it is speculated that the lipophilicity of drugs contributes to the pharmacokinetic properties of dihydropyridines oxidizing with intestinal CYP3A. On the other hand, some dihydropyridines showed values that were distant from the linear regression in Figure 13. This observation possibly suggests that alternative factors other than CYP3A, such as drug transporters in the intestine, may be involved in the interactions. It has been reported that concomitant intake of GFJ causes an increase in the plasma concentration of P-glycoprotein substrates such as cyclosporine (Edwards, 1999) and a decrease in the plasma concentration of organic anion transporting peptide (OATP) substrates such as fexofenadine (Dresser, 2005). ALOGPs were considered to be the most appropriate algorithm to assess the interactions between the three types of predicted logP values examined in this study because they showed the best correlation. ALOGPs were used to predict the extent of GFJ interactions with dihydropyridines, which has not been reported to date. As a result, lercanidipine and niguldipine (ALOGPs: 6.42 and 6.27, respectively) were estimated to be high-risk drugs showing a predictive increase of 300% in the AUC with GFJ intake. Alternatively, it was suggested that aranidipine and nilvadipine (ALOGPs: 2.71 and 2.97, respectively) which are used in Japanese clinical practice, are relatively safe drugs comparable to nifedipine, which has a predicted AUC increase with GFJ of about 150%. The adequacy of these prognostics has yet to be demonstrated in terms of clinical trials, although the structural analyses in this study will be useful to predict the harmfulness of drugs in interactions with GFJ.

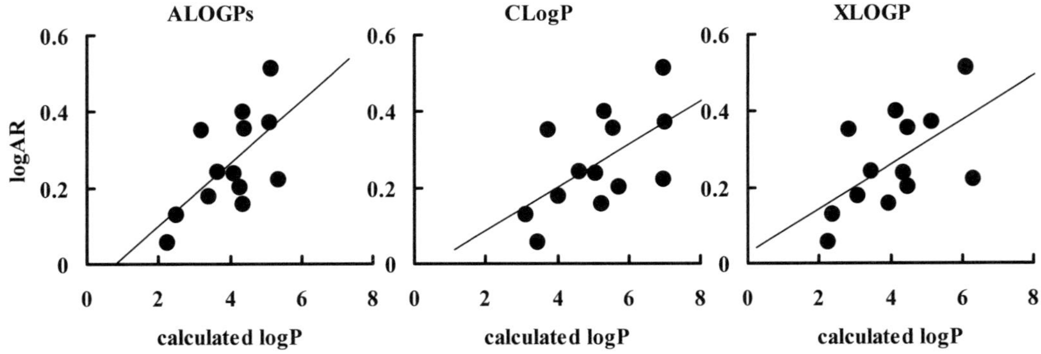

Lines are drawn with the least-squares approach.
AR: AUC ratio.
This figure was cited from the literature (Uesawa & Mohri, 2008c).

Fig. 13. Relationship Between Calculated LogP Values of Dihydropyridine Derivatives and the Corresponding Logarithmic AUC Ratios in Clinical Trials with GFJ Consumption.

2.6 Elimination of interacting components in GFJ

We found that BG and DHB in GFJ were unstable at high temperatures (Uesawa & Mohri, 2006). It is therefore proposed that the heat treatment of GFJ might serve as the basis for the removal of interactive FCs and thus the elimination of potential drug interactions. Furthermore, GFJ samples after heat treatment under various conditions, including various concentrations of FCs, are still useful for elucidating the functions of FCs in drug interactions. With such a background, we studied the effect of incubation at various temperatures on the concentrations of FCs in GFJ, and the actions of the GFJ samples on the drug interactions *in vitro* and *in vivo*. BG and DHB showed a consistent decrease during treatment at 95°C for 1 hr (Figure 14). Interestingly, the concentration of BT in GFJ was reversely increased in this condition. The increment of BT in GFJ rose to 14.1 μM after 60 min of treatment. At 4 and 37°C, each FC concentration did not almost change during incubation for 60 min (Figure 14). At 62, 72, and 95°C, concentrations of BG and DHB decreased in a temperature-dependent manner. The remainders of BG and DHB at 95°C for 60 min were 3.14 and 0.163 μM, respectively. On the other hand, the concentration of BT at 95°C for 60 min was 64.8 μM.

2.6.1 Inhibition of CYP3A activities

The testosterone 6β-hydroxylation rate was 2.14 nmol/min/mg protein in human liver microsomes; 10% of GFJ in the reaction mixture decreased the oxidation activity to 0.303 nmol/min/mg protein (14.1 % of the control, Figure 15). Treatment of GFJ at 95°C invalidated the inhibitory effect of GFJ by heat treatment in a time-dependent manner. The testosterone 6β-hydroxylation rate with GFJ heat-treated at 95°C for 60 min (HGJ) was 0.617 nmol/min/mg protein (28.8 % of the control). The remaining concentrations of BG and DHB, the important constituents in GFJ for drug interactions (section 1.3), in HGJ were 3.13 and 0.16 μM, respectively. On the other hand, BT, which does not contribute to CYP3A inhibition in GFJ, was increased to 64.8 μM in HGJ (Figure. 13). It was expected from these results that the CYP3A inhibitory effect and the pharmacokinetic interactions of GFJ would disappear as a result of heat treatment. Then, testosterone 6β-hydroxylation with human liver microsomes and GFJ treated at 95°C were measured in order to investigate the effect of the heating on CYP3A oxidation. As a result, the turnover rate of 6β-hydroxylation of testosterone decreased as the duration of heat treatment increased (Figure 15). The testosterone 6β-hydroxylation rates were negatively related to the concentrations of BG and DHB in GFJ samples treated at 95°C. These observations suggest that the lower amounts of BG and DHB in GFJ due to heating at 95°C controlled the inhibition of testosterone 6β-hydroxylation with GFJ. No study of inhibition of the CYP3A metabolism with FC-free GFJ has been reported. In this study, the remaining activities of CYP3A in the microsomal reactions with GFJ and HGJ were 14.1% and 28.8%, respectively, compared with the reaction without GFJ. It is believed that the 14.7% difference between the results with HGJ and GFJ stem from the net inhibition with BG and DHB in this condition. BG and DHB have structures constructed with BT, the simplest FC in citrus fruits, and isoprene side chains combined through the fifth oxygen atom of BT (Figure 2). It was reported that BG and DHB decrease oxidation for the drugs with mechanism-based inhibition of CYP3A expressed in small intestinal epithelial cells (Ameer & Weintraub, 1997). On the other hand, BT did not inhibit CYP3A activities in microsomes from humans and rats (Mohri & Uesawa, 2001a; Row, 2006).

2.6.2 Effects of HGJ on nifedipine pharmacokinetics

It was shown that HGJ produced a CYP3A-inhibitory effect of 71% in comparison with untreated GFJ. Therefore the effects of HGJ on nifedipine pharmacokinetics in rats were evaluated in vivo. We have shown, in earlier studies, that the AUC of nifedipine is significantly increased by the intraduodenal administration of GFJ but not of orange juice, sweetie juice, or saline (Mohri, 2000; Mohri & Uesawa, 2001a; Uesawa & Mohri, 2005). These results suggest that GFJ caused increased gastrointestinal absorption of nifedipine in rats. It was thought that nifedipine oxidation by CYP3A in the intestinal mucosa was inhibited by GFJ administration. Actually, our rat studies with small intestinal microsomes (Mohri & Uesawa, 2001b) indicated that BG and DHB contribute to the inhibition of nifedipine oxidation in rat small intestine (Mohri & Uesawa, 2001a). These observations in rats are very similar to those in humans (Lown et al., 1997). These observations suggest that evaluation using rats is useful for predicting drug-food interactions. Therefore the effect of HGJ administration on nifedipine pharmacokinetics using rats was investigated in this study. Injection of HGJ into the duodenum 30 min before nifedipine administration did not affect the plasma concentration/time profile of nifedipine (Figure 16). On the other hand, the AUC and C_{max} were significantly increased in the GFJ-preadministered group compared with the HGJ-administered group. These observations show that the administration of HGJ, unlike that of GFJ, probably does not increase the small intestinal absorption of nifedipine. The results also suggest that inhibitory contents of CYP3A in HGJ, as observed in the in vitro experiments, because of the disappearance of BG and DHB in HGJ, do not contribute pharmacokinetic interactions between nifedipine and GFJ. Mechanism-based inhibitors such as BG and DHB may be able to reduce the activity of CYP3A in the intestinal tract effectively (Ameer & Weintraub, 1997). In fact, unlike GFJ, naringin, a potent, but not mechanism-based inhibitor of CYP3A (Guengerich & Kim, 1990), has been reported not to increase the availability of nisoldipine in humans (Bailey et al., 1993b).

These investigations clearly showed the contributions of FCs on drug interactions with GFJ in *in vitro* and *in vivo* experiments using GFJ samples, eliminated BG and DHB following high temperature treatments. Furthermore, these observations may develop as fundamental knowledge to create "drinkable GFJ" for patients receiving medications that induce interactions with GFJ. In the previous report, we showed that sweetie juice did not have a significant effect on nifedipine pharmacokinetics in rats (Uesawa & Mohri, 2005). The concentrations of BG and DHB in the sweetie juice used in the study were 1.6 and 0.51 μM, respectively. In other words, low FC concentrations such as that in sweetie juice and HGJ hardly relate to drug bioavailability. Examination of the respective threshold concentrations of the FCs is important in terms of pharmacokinetics in order to ensure the quality of the GFJ from which FCs have been removed. On the other hand, heat treatment at 95 °C in the present basic study seems to have a detrimental effect on the taste, flavor and nutrients of GFJ. However, it might be possible to develop GFJ processing methods with lower temperatures thereby avoiding these problems, as, the concentrations of BG and DHB in GFJ are low at 62 °C. In addition, understanding the thermal decomposition mechanism of FCs may enable the selection of effective low-temperature catalysts. Although it is necessary to examine the heating condition, we presumed that the results of the heat treatment of GFJ will contribute to the development of practical research on the prevention of drug interactions, and may contribute to resolving this problem in clinical settings. This study offers a new method that is applicable in research on drug interaction with various food and drinks.

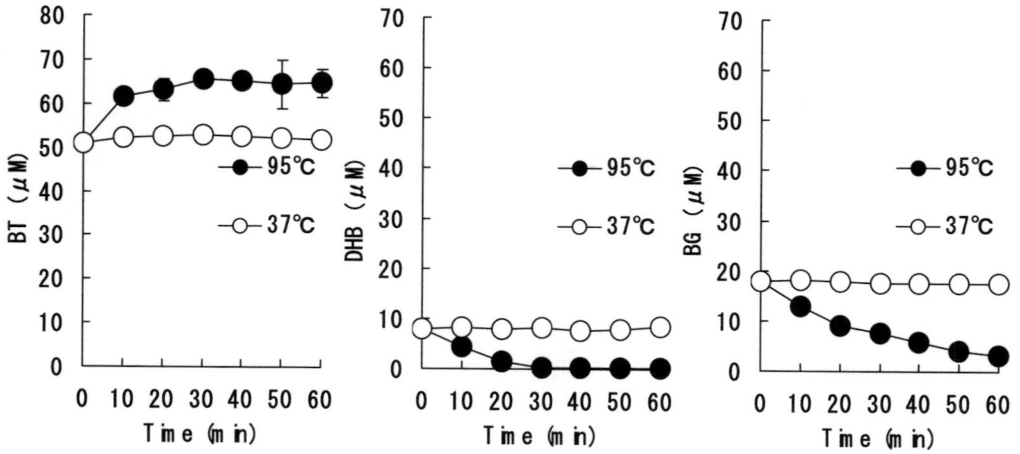

The concentrations were determined in duplicate as described under Materials and Methods. Each point and vertical bar represents the mean and range. This figure was cited from the literature (Uesawa & Mohri, 2006).

Fig. 14. BT, DHB, and BG concentrations in the GFJ treated at 37°C and 95°C for 0, 10, 20, 30, 40, 50, and 60min.

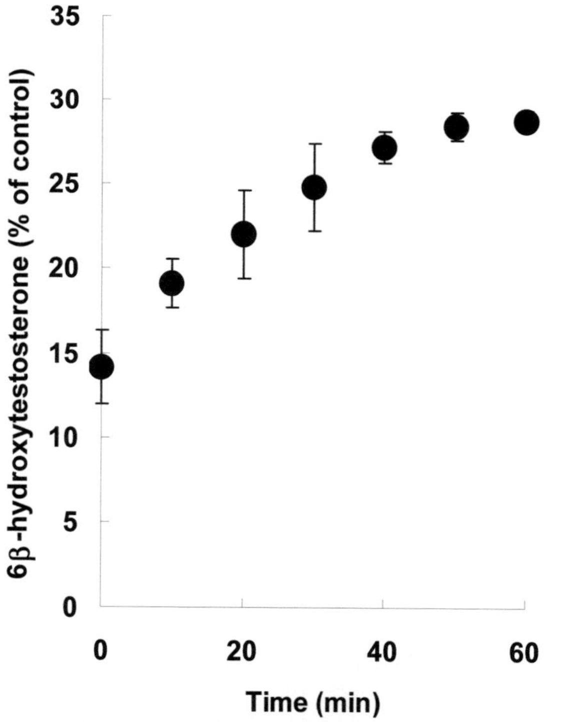

The control mixture included no GFJ. Each point and vertical bar represents the mean and S.D. (n=3). This figure was cited from the literature (Uesawa & Mohri, 2006).

Fig. 15. 6β-oxidation rates of testosterone with human liver microsomes and the GFJ treated at 95°C for 0, 10, 20, 30, 40, 50, and 60 min.

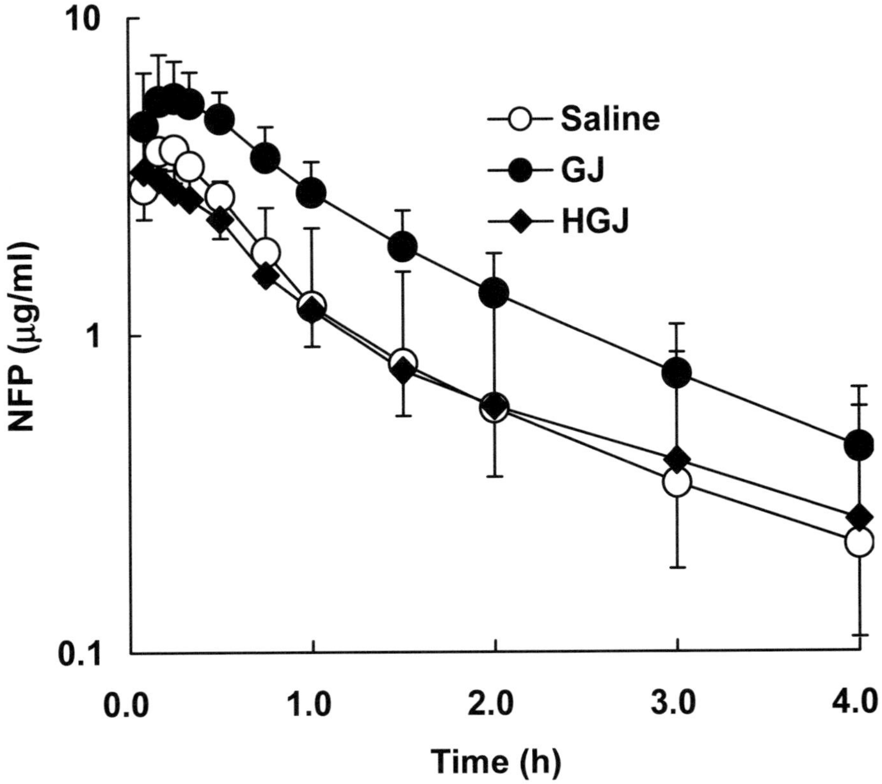

Dose of nifedipine=3mg/kg. Five rats were used in each group. Each point and vertical bar represents the mean and S.D. (n=5). This figure was cited from the literature (Uesawa & Mohri, 2006).

Fig. 16. Plasma concentration-time curves for nifedipine after i.d. administration of nifedipine 30 min after administration of 2 mL of saline, GFJ, and HGJ to the duodenum.

2.7 Variation of concentrations of furanocoumarin derivatives in GFJ brands

2.7.1 Drug-interaction potentials among different brands of GFJ

We discovered that heat treatment of GFJ decreased concentrations of furanocoumarin derivatives, bergamottin and 6',7'-dihydroxybergamottin, depending on the temperature and the treatment period, thereby causing the inhibitory effect on CYP3A to decrease and the pharmacokinetic interaction potential to disappear (Section 1-6). These findings suggest that heat treatment of GFJ may be applicable in the evaluation of GFJ-drug interactions from furanocoumarins, suggesting that the decrease in the CYP3A inhibitory potential of GFJ by the heat treatment was related to the concentrations of furanocoumarins present in GFJ. In this section, variations in the drug-interactions among 21 different brands of GFJ were estimated using heat treatment to analyze the potentials of furanocoumarin-caused CYP3A-inhibitions (Uesawa & Mohri, 2008b). Heat treatment of the GFJ at 95 °C for 1h was utilized to degrade the furanocoumarins. Initial velocity of testosterone 6β-oxidation using human liver microsomes was determined as an indicator of the CYP3A activities. The initial rates of CYP3A dependent testosterone 6β-oxidation in human liver microsomes were measured with various brands of GFJ and heat-treated GFJ (HGJ). As a result, when compared with the corresponding brand of untreated GFJ, all brands of HGJs indicated significantly lower efficacy in the inhibition of the CYP3A oxidation, except for one brand that showed no significant change (Figure 17). The inhibitory effects of untreated GFJ and HGJ ranged from 54.2 to 85.9 % and from 25.0 to 71.1%, respectively. The differences between the two, caused by the loss of furanocoumarins in heating, were defined as net potentials of furanocoumarin-induced CYP3A inhibitions (FCIs) and expressed as percentages compared with the control velocity in a 6β - hydroxytestosterone - production reaction without GFJ (Figure 18). The results show that FCIs ranged from 4.0 to 35.9%.

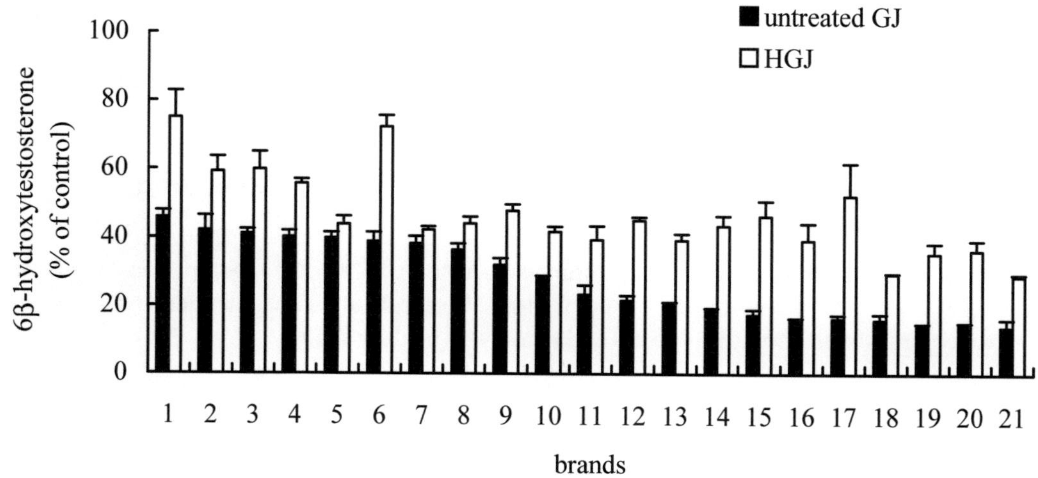

The control mixture included no GFJ. Each point and vertical bar represents the mean and S.D. (n=3). This figure was cited from the literature (Uesawa & Mohri, 2008b).

Fig. 17. 6β-oxidation rates of testosterone with human liver microsomes and untreated GFJ or HGJ.

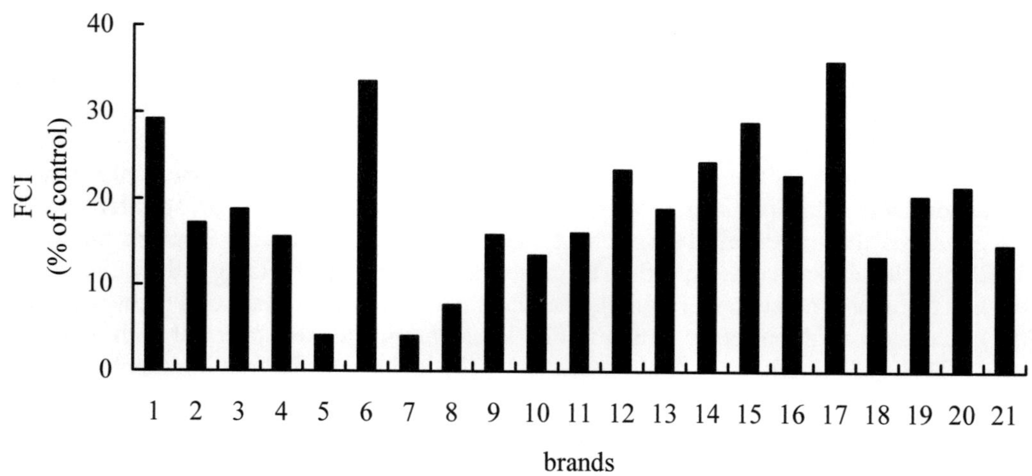

This figure was cited from the literature (Uesawa & Mohri, 2008b).

Fig. 18. FCI values in each GFJ sample.

The component inhibitory potentials eliminated by the heat treatment of GFJ may be able to reflect the action *in vivo*. The results indicate that heat treatment could be useful in evaluating the potencies of GFJs in the drug interactions caused by furanocoumarins. It is believed that the *in vitro* evaluation systems using only untreated GFJ do not properly reflect the GFJ - drug interactions *in vivo* because these interactions are induced by furanocoumarin derivatives such as bergamottin and 6',7 '- dihydroxybergamottin in GFJ. Figure 17 and 18 show that order of each bland on the interaction potential estimated by FCI is not necessarily corresponding to the case estimated by only untreated GFJ. Therefore, we suggest that the inhibition potential of GFJ may be estimated by subtracting the microsomal CYP3A activity with HGJ from those activities obtained with the corresponding untreated GFJ. It is anticipated that the technical measurements of the GFJ-drug interaction potentials using FCI established in the present study, may be an effective method to identify the intensity of GFJ in the interactions.

3. Citrus juice interactions related with the decrease of plasma drug concentrations

Recently, citrus juices such as GFJ and orange juice can prevent the intestinal absorption of some β-blockers. As a result of this type of interactions, plasma concentrations of drugs are decreased. In this section, this type of interaction will be described.

3.1 Antihypertensive drugs related with the citrus juice interactions

In addition to increasing drug absorption with GFJ, citrus juices such as GFJ and orange juice can also prevent the intestinal absorption of drugs. For example, the intestinal absorption of fexofenadine, a third-generation antihistamine, is inhibited by GFJ, orange juice, and apple juice (Dresser, 2002). Furthermore, GFJ and orange juice also inhibit absorption of the ß-blocking agents, celiprolol (Lilja, 2003, 2004), atenolol (Lilja, 2005b), acebutolol (Lilja, 2005a), and talinolol (Schwarz, 2005).

3.2 Mechanism of the citrus juice interactions

It was reported that the citrus juice interactions are caused by inhibition of drug-transporting ability of intestinal organic anion transporting polypeptide (OATP) with contents in citrus juices. Fexofenadine is taken up by intestinal epithelial cells via OATP, which is expressed on the apical membrane, in the first step of absorption into general circulation from intestinal lumen (Dresser et al., 2002, 2005; Nozawa, 2004). Interestingly, GFJ enhances the intestinal absorption of talinolol in rats, putatively through inhibiting MDR1 activity and decreasing efflux from epithelial cells (Spahn-Langguth & Langguth, 2001). In humans, however, GFJ inhibits the intestinal absorption of talinolol (Schwarz et al., 2005). These observations suggest that in GFJ interactions with substrates of both of MDR1 and OATP, OATP uptake may dominate MDR1 efflux in humans but not in rodents.

3.3 Citrus juice components involved in drug interactions

Naringin, the major ingredient in GFJ, blocks the uptake of fexofenadine by the intestinal cells (Bailey, 2007). Hesperidin, a major component of orange juice, also inhibits intestinal absorption of celiprolol (Uesawa & Mohri, 2008a). Hesperidin is a flavonoid glycoside with a similar molecular structure to naringin. Hesperidin and naringin both inhibit the transport of OATP1A2 (Bailey et al., 2007), which mediates the intestinal uptake and systemic accessibility of ß-blockers, providing a mechanism for inhibiting absorption (Bailey et al., 2007).

In this section, our findings related with demonstration of a causal ingredient of the pharmacokinetic interaction between orange juice and celiprolol. It has been reported that the bioavailability of celiprolol is decreased by interaction with orange juice as well as GFJ because of inhibition of intestinal absorption of the drug (Lilja et al., 2004). We attempted to characterize this interaction by means of pharmacokinetic experiments with rats. Figure 19 shows pharmacokinetic profiles of plasma celiprolol levels when celiprolol with water (control), orange juice, and hesperidin solution were injected into the rat duodenum. However, under the abundant period of the elimination phase, especially for the orange juice group, the pharmacokinetic parameters were calculated in the period for descriptive purposes as well as other groups. AUC of celiprolol in the orange juice group was significantly decreased by 75.3 % compared with the control group. This observation corresponds with results in humans in which the AUC of celiprolol decreased by 83 %. It has been known in detail that when fexofenadine is taken with grapefruit or orange juice, both plasma concentration and AUC are decreased, as in the case of celiprolol. It has been reported that naringin, a major ingredient in GFJ, was the cause of the pharmacokinetic interaction between GFJ and fexofenadine (Bailey et al., 2007). Hesperidin, a major component of orange juice, is a flavonoid glycoside with an appearance and molecular structure similar to that of naringin. It has been demonstrated that hesperidin as well as naringin inhibit the transport of OATP1A2, an intestinal transporter related to the absorption of fexofenadine (Bailey et al., 2007). OATP1A2 probably facilitates the intestinal uptake and systemic accessibility of a broad battery of orally administered medications (Lee, 2005; Glaeser, 2007). Rat intestinal oatp3 is an orthologue of human OATP1A2 (Dresser et al., 2002). Although the mechanism of inhibition of celiprolol absorption by orange juice is unknown, flavonoids possibly contribute to the interaction because celiprolol undergoes inhibition with both orange juice and GFJ in the same way as fexofenadine. In fact, hesperidin as well as naringin affected significantly the uptake of fexofenadine by rat oatp3 (Dresser et al., 2002). We therefore designed our study with rats with the intention of identifying the role of hesperidin in orange juice in the interaction with celiprolol. As a result of the administration of celiprolol with hesperidin, significant decreases in AUC were observed compared with control, as also in the case of concomitant orange juice administration. On the other hand, the AUC in the hesperidin group was not significantly different from that in the orange juice group. These results demonstrate that hesperidin in orange juice contributes to the interaction observed. Inhibition of the celiprolol transporting pathway by hesperidin in the intestine is a possible mechanisms as is the case with fexofenadine - orange juice interaction. Furthermore, physicochemical effects such as binding and degradation of celiprolol with hesperidin might also contribute to the reduction in plasma concentrations due to decreased solubility and absolute amount of the drug in the intestinal duct. Initial decrementation of the celiprolol concentration in plasma by the coadministration of orange juice was greater than that due to hesperidin (Figure 19). In the rats receiving orange juice but not hesperidin, Tmax was also elongated significantly compared with controls. These observations suggest that a component or components of orange juice other than hesperidin may also contribute to variations in the absorption kinetics of celiprolol.

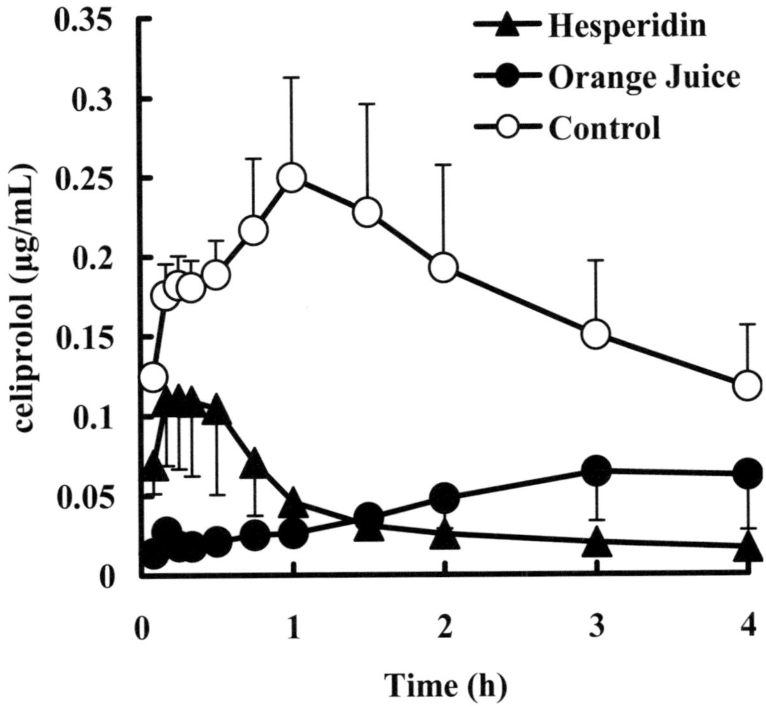

Dose of celiprolol was 5 mg/kg body weight. Each point and vertical bar represents the mean and S.E., respectively (n=4 - 5). This figure was cited from the literature (Uesawa & Mohri, 2008a).

Fig. 19. Plasma concentration-time curves for celiprolol after it was administered into the duodenum of rats with water (control, white circle), orange juice (black circle) and 207.7 μg/mL hesperidin aqueous solution (black triangle).

4. Conclusion

Accumulated knowledge of pharmacokinetic interactions of antihypertensive drugs with citrus juices was mentioned in this chapter. Furthermore, characteristics and mechanisms of the interactions were described with the latest results in the research studies. Drug-citrus juice interactions are a complicated phenomenon, with increasing and decreasing drug concentrations in plasma which is dependent on the combinations of drugs and juices. However, I believe that applicable instruction based on an understanding of the mechanisms for patients undergoing pharmaceutical therapies, will be useful. This will enable them to avoid such interactions.

5. References

Ameer, B. and Weintraub, RA. (1997). Drug interactions with grapefruit juice. *Clin Pharmacokinet*, Vol.33, No.2, pp.103-121, ISSN 0312-5963

Azuma, J., Yamamoto, I., Watase, T., Seto, Y., Tanaka, T., Katoh, M., Orii, Y., Tanigawa, T., Yoshikawa, K., Terajima, S. and Matsuki, T. (1996). Effects of grapefruit juice on the pharmacokinetics of the calcium antagonists nifedipine and nisoldipine. *Jpn*

Pharmacol Ther, Vol.24, No.2, pp.461-470, ISSN Japanese Pharmacology and Therapeutics

Baarnhielm, C., Skanberg, I. and Borg, KO. (1984). Cytochrome P-450-dependent oxidation of felodipine--a 1,4-dihydropyridine--to the corresponding pyridine. *Xenobiotica*, Vol.14, No.9, pp.719-726, ISSN 0049-8254

Bailey, DG., Arnold, JM., Bend, JR., Tran, LT. and Spence, JD. (1995). Grapefruit juice-felodipine interaction: reproducibility and characterization with the extended release drug formulation. *Br J Clin Pharmacol*, Vol.40, No.2, pp.135-140,

Bailey, DG., Arnold, JM., Munoz, C. and Spence, JD. (1993a). Grapefruit juice--felodipine interaction: mechanism, predictability, and effect of naringin. *Clin Pharmacol Ther*, Vol.53, No.6, pp.637-642,

Bailey, DG., Arnold, JM., Strong, HA., Munoz, C. and Spence, JD. (1993b). Effect of grapefruit juice and naringin on nisoldipine pharmacokinetics. *Clin Pharmacol Ther*, Vol.54, No.6, pp.589-594, ISSN 0009-9236

Bailey, DG., Bend, JR., Arnold, JM., Tran, LT. and Spence, JD. (1996). Erythromycin-felodipine interaction: magnitude, mechanism, and comparison with grapefruit juice. *Clin Pharmacol Ther*, Vol.60, No.1, pp.25-33,

Bailey, DG., Dresser, GK. and Bend, JR. (2003). Bergamottin, lime juice, and red wine as inhibitors of cytochrome P450 3A4 activity: comparison with grapefruit juice. *Clin Pharmacol Ther*, Vol.73, No.6, pp.529-537,

Bailey, DG., Dresser, GK., Kreeft, JH., Munoz, C., Freeman, DJ. and Bend, JR. (2000). Grapefruit-felodipine interaction: effect of unprocessed fruit and probable active ingredients. *Clin Pharmacol Ther*, Vol.68, No.5, pp.468-477,

Bailey, DG., Dresser, GK., Leake, BF. and Kim, RB. (2007). Naringin is a major and selective clinical inhibitor of organic anion-transporting polypeptide 1A2 (OATP1A2) in grapefruit juice. *Clin Pharmacol Ther*, Vol.81, No.4, pp.495-502,

Bailey, DG., Kreeft, JH., Munoz, C., Freeman, DJ. and Bend, JR. (1998). Grapefruit juice-felodipine interaction: effect of naringin and 6',7'-dihydroxybergamottin in humans. *Clin Pharmacol Ther*, Vol.64, No.3, pp.248-256, ISSN 0009-9236

Bailey, DG., Spence, JD., Edgar, B., Bayliff, CD. and Arnold, JM. (1989). Ethanol enhances the hemodynamic effects of felodipine. *Clin Invest Med*, Vol.12, No.6, pp.357-362, ISSN 0147-958X

Bailey, DG., Spence, JD., Munoz, C. and Arnold, JM. (1991). Interaction of citrus juices with felodipine and nifedipine. *Lancet*, Vol.337, No.8736, pp.268-269, ISSN 0140-6736

Cantelli-Forti, G., Guerra, MC., Barbaro, AM., Hrelia, P., Biagi, GL. and Borea, PA. (1986). Relationship between lipophilic character and urinary excretion of nitroimidazoles and nitrothiazoles in rats. *J Med Chem*, Vol.29, No.4, pp.555-561, ISSN 0022-2623

Chou, JT. and Jurs, PC. (1979). Computer-assisted computation of partition coefficients from molecular structures using fragment constants. *J Chem Inf Comput Sci*, Vol.19, No.3, pp.172-178, ISSN 0095-2338

Dresser, GK., Bailey, DG., Leake, BF., Schwarz, UI., Dawson, PA., Freeman, DJ. and Kim, RB. (2002). Fruit juices inhibit organic anion transporting polypeptide-mediated drug uptake to decrease the oral availability of fexofenadine. *Clin Pharmacol Ther*, Vol.71, No.1, pp.11-20,

Dresser, GK., Kim, RB. and Bailey, DG. (2005). Effect of grapefruit juice volume on the reduction of fexofenadine bioavailability: possible role of organic anion transporting polypeptides. *Clin Pharmacol Ther*, Vol.77, No.3, pp.170-177,

Eagling, VA., Profit, L. and Back, DJ. (1999). Inhibition of the CYP3A4-mediated metabolism and P-glycoprotein-mediated transport of the HIV-1 protease inhibitor saquinavir by grapefruit juice components. *Br J Clin Pharmacol*, Vol.48, No.4, pp.543-552,

Edgar, B., Bailey, D., Bergstrand, R., Johnsson, G. and Regårdh, CG. (1992). Acute effects of drinking grapefruit juice on the pharmacokinetics and dynamics of felodipine--and its potential clinical relevance. *Eur J Clin Pharmacol*, Vol.42, No.3, pp.313-317, ISSN 0031-6970

Edwards, DJ., Fitzsimmons, ME., Schuetz, EG., Yasuda, K., Ducharme, MP., Warbasse, LH., Woster, PM., Schuetz, JD. and Watkins, P. (1999). 6',7'-Dihydroxybergamottin in grapefruit juice and Seville orange juice: effects on cyclosporine disposition, enterocyte CYP3A4, and P-glycoprotein. *Clin Pharmacol Ther*, Vol.65, No.3, pp.237-244,

Fuhr, U., Klittich, K. and Staib, AH. (1993). Inhibitory effect of grapefruit juice and its bitter principal, naringenin, on CYP1A2 dependent metabolism of caffeine in man. *Br J Clin Pharmacol*, Vol.35, No.4, pp.431-436,

Fuhr, U., Maier-Bruggemann, A., Blume, H., Muck, W., Unger, S., Kuhlmann, J., Huschka, C., Zaigler, M., Rietbrock, S. and Staib, AH. (1998). Grapefruit juice increases oral nimodipine bioavailability. *Int J Clin Pharmacol Ther*, Vol.36, No.3, pp.126-132, ISSN 0946-1965

Fujioka, T., Furumi, K., Fujii, H., Okabe, H., Mihashi, K., Nakano, Y., Matsunaga, H., Katano, M. and Mori, M. (1999). Antiproliferative constituents from umbelliferae plants. V. A new furanocoumarin and falcarindiol furanocoumarin ethers from the root of Angelica japonica. *Chem Pharm Bull (Tokyo)*, Vol.47, No.1, pp.96-100, ISSN 0009-2363

Girennavar, B., Poulose, SM., Jayaprakasha, GK., Bhat, NG. and Patil, BS. (2006). Furocoumarins from grapefruit juice and their effect on human CYP 3A4 and CYP 1B1 isoenzymes. *Bioorg Med Chem*, Vol.14, No.8, pp.2606-2612,

Glaeser, H., Bailey, DG., Dresser, GK., Gregor, JC., Schwarz, UI., McGrath, JS., Jolicoeur, E., Lee, W., Leake, BF., Tirona, RG. and Kim, RB. (2007). Intestinal drug transporter expression and the impact of grapefruit juice in humans. *Clin Pharmacol Ther*, Vol.81, No.3, pp.362-370,

Goosen, TC., Cillié, D., Bailey, DG., Yu, C., He, K., Hollenberg, PF., Woster, PM., Cohen, L., Williams, JA., Rheeders, M. and Dijkstra, HP. (2004). Bergamottin contribution to the grapefruit juice-felodipine interaction and disposition in humans. *Clin Pharmacol Ther*, Vol.76, No.6, pp.607-617,

Grenier, J., Fradette, C., Morelli, G., Merritt, GJ., Vranderick, M. and Ducharme, MP. (2006). Pomelo juice, but not cranberry juice, affects the pharmacokinetics of cyclosporine in humans. *Clin Pharmacol Ther*, Vol.79, No.3, pp.255-262,

Guengerich, FP. and Kim, DH. (1990). In vitro inhibition of dihydropyridine oxidation and aflatoxin B1 activation in human liver microsomes by naringenin and other flavonoids. *Carcinogenesis*, Vol.11, No.12, pp.2275-2279,

Guo, LQ., Taniguchi, M., Xiao, YQ., Baba, K., Ohta, T. and Yamazoe, Y. (2000). Inhibitory effect of natural furanocoumarins on human microsomal cytochrome P450 3A activity. *Japanese Journal of Pharmacology*, Vol.82, No.2, pp.122-129, ISSN 0021-5198

Hashimoto, K., Shirafuji, T., Sekino, H., Matsuoka, O., Sekino, H., Onnagawa, O., Okamoto, T., Kudo, S. and Azuma, J. (1998). Interaction of citrus juices with pranidipine, a new 1,4-dihydropyridine calcium antagonist, in healthy subjects. *Eur J Clin Pharmacol*, Vol.54, No.9-10, pp.753-760, ISSN 0031-6970

He, K., Iyer, KR., Hayes, RN., Sinz, MW., Woolf, TF. and Hollenberg, PF. (1998). Inactivation of cytochrome P450 3A4 by bergamottin, a component of grapefruit juice. *Chem Res Toxicol*, Vol.11, No.4, pp.252-259, ISSN 0893-228X

Hirashima, H., Uchida, N., Fukuzawa, I., Ishigaki, S., Uchida, E. and Yasuhara, H. (2006). Effect of a single glass of grapefruit juice on the apparent oral bioavailability of the dihydropyridine calcium channel antagonist, azelnidipine, in healthy japanese volunteers. *Jpn J Clin Pharmacol Ther*, Vol.37, No.3, pp.127-133, ISSN Jpn J Clin Pharmacol Ther

Ho, PC., Ghose, K., Saville, D. and Wanwimolruk, S. (2000). Effect of grapefruit juice on pharmacokinetics and pharmacodynamics of verapamil enantiomers in healthy volunteers. *Eur J Clin Pharmacol*, Vol.56, No.9-10, pp.693-698, ISSN 0031-6970

Houston, JB., Upshall, DG. and Bridges, JW. (1975). Further studies using carbamate esters as model compounds to investigate the role of lipophilicity in the gastrointestinal absorption of foreign compounds. *J Pharmacol Exp Ther*, Vol.195, No.1, pp.67-72,

Josefsson, M., Zackrisson, AL. and Ahlner, J. (1996). Effect of grapefruit juice on the pharmacokinetics of amlodipine in healthy volunteers. *Eur J Clin Pharmacol*, Vol.51, No.2, pp.189-193, ISSN 0031-6970

Kane, GC. and Lipsky, JJ. (2000). Drug-grapefruit juice interactions. *Mayo Clin Proc*, Vol.75, No.9, pp.933-942, ISSN 0025-6196

Kiehs, K., Hansch, C. and Moore, L. (1966). The role of hydrophobic bonding in the binding of organic compounds by bovine hemoglobin. *Biochemistry*, Vol.5, No.8, pp.2602-2605, ISSN 0006-2960

Kim, KH. (1991). Quantitative structure-activity relationships of the metabolism of drugs by uridine diphosphate glucuronosyltransferase. *J Pharm Sci*, Vol.80, No.10, pp.966-970, ISSN 0022-3549

Lee, W., Glaeser, H., Smith, LH., Roberts, RL., Moeckel, GW., Gervasini, G., Leake, BF. and Kim, RB. (2005). Polymorphisms in human organic anion-transporting polypeptide 1A2 (OATP1A2): implications for altered drug disposition and central nervous system drug entry. *J Biol Chem*, Vol.280, No.10, pp.9610-9617,

Lewis, DF. (2000). Structural characteristics of human P450s involved in drug metabolism: QSARs and lipophilicity profiles. *Toxicology*, Vol.144, No.1-3, pp.197-203, ISSN 0300-483X

Lilja, JJ., Backman, JT., Laitila, J., Luurila, H. and Neuvonen, PJ. (2003). Itraconazole increases but grapefruit juice greatly decreases plasma concentrations of celiprolol. *Clin Pharmacol Ther*, Vol.73, No.3, pp.192-198,

Lilja, JJ., Juntti-Patinen, L. and Neuvonen, PJ. (2004). Orange juice substantially reduces the bioavailability of the beta-adrenergic-blocking agent celiprolol. *Clin Pharmacol Ther*, Vol.75, No.3, pp.184-190,

Lilja, JJ., Kivisto, KT. and Neuvonen, PJ. (1998). Grapefruit juice-simvastatin interaction: effect on serum concentrations of simvastatin, simvastatin acid, and HMG-CoA reductase inhibitors. *Clin Pharmacol Ther*, Vol.64, No.5, pp.477-483, ISSN 0009-9236

Lilja, JJ., Raaska, K. and Neuvonen, PJ. (2005a). Effects of grapefruit juice on the pharmacokinetics of acebutolol. *Br J Clin Pharmacol*, Vol.60, No.6, pp.659-663,

Lilja, JJ., Raaska, K. and Neuvonen, PJ. (2005b). Effects of orange juice on the pharmacokinetics of atenolol. *Eur J Clin Pharmacol*, Vol.61, No.5-6, pp.337-340, ISSN 0031-6970

Lown, KS., Bailey, DG., Fontana, RJ., Janardan, SK., Adair, CH., Fortlage, LA., Brown, MB., Guo, W. and Watkins, PB. (1997). Grapefruit juice increases felodipine oral availability in humans by decreasing intestinal CYP3A protein expression. *J Clin Invest*, Vol.99, No.10, pp.2545-2553, ISSN 0021-9738

Lundahl, J., Regårdh, CG., Edgar, B. and Johnsson, G. (1995). Relationship between time of intake of grapefruit juice and its effect on pharmacokinetics and pharmacodynamics of felodipine in healthy subjects. *Eur J Clin Pharmacol*, Vol.49, No.1-2, pp.61-67, ISSN 0031-6970

Lundahl, J., Regårdh, CG., Edgar, B. and Johnsson, G. (1997). Effects of grapefruit juice ingestion--pharmacokinetics and haemodynamics of intravenously and orally administered felodipine in healthy men. *Eur J Clin Pharmacol*, Vol.52, No.2, pp.139-145, ISSN 0031-6970

Malhotra, S., Bailey, DG., Paine, MF. and Watkins, PB. (2001). Seville orange juice-felodipine interaction: comparison with dilute grapefruit juice and involvement of furocoumarins. *Clin Pharmacol Ther*, Vol.69, No.1, pp.14-23,

Mimura, G., Jinnouchi, T. and Nanno, S. (1998). Studies on interactions between grapefruit juice and calcium chanel blockers (4): effects of grapefruit juice on pharmacokinetics of efonidipine hydrochloride. *The Japanese Journal of Constitutional Medicine*, Vol.60, No.1, pp.23-37, ISSN The Japanese Journal of Constitutional Medicine

Mimura, G., Nanno, S. and Ohshita, T. (2000). Studies on effects of grapefruit on pharmacokinetics of efonidipine hydrochloride. *The Japanese Journal of Constitutional Medicine*, Vol.62, No.1, pp.44-51, ISSN The Japanese Journal of Constitutional Medicine

Mohri, K. and Uesawa, Y. (2001a). Effects of furanocoumarin derivatives in grapefruit juice on nifedipine pharmacokinetics in rats. *Pharm Res*, Vol.18, No.2, pp.177-182, ISSN 0724-8741

Mohri, K. and Uesawa, Y. (2001b). Enzymatic activities in the microsomes prepared from rat small intestinal epithelial cells by differential procedures. *Pharm Res*, Vol.18, No.8, pp.1232-1236, ISSN 0724-8741

Mohri, K., Uesawa, Y. and Sagawa, K. (2000). Effects of long-term grapefruit juice ingestion on nifedipine pharmacokinetics: induction of rat hepatic P-450 by grapefruit juice. *Drug Metab Dispos*, Vol.28, No.4, pp.482-486,

Nozawa, T., Imai, K., Nezu, J., Tsuji, A. and Tamai, I. (2004). Functional characterization of pH-sensitive organic anion transporting polypeptide OATP-B in human. *J Pharmacol Exp Ther*, Vol.308, No.2, pp.438-445,

Ohnishi, A., Ohtani, H. and Sawada, Y. (2006). Major determinant factors of the extent of interaction between grapefruit juice and calcium channel antagonists. *Br J Clin Pharmacol*, Vol.62, No.2, pp.196-199, ISSN 0306-5251

Ohtani, M., Kawabata, S., Kariya, S., Uchino, K., Itou, K., Kotaki, H., Kasuyama, K., Morikawa, A., Seo, I. and Nishida, N. (2002). Effect of grapefruit pulp on the pharmacokinetics of the dihydropyridine calcium antagonists nifedipine and nisoldipine. *Yakugaku Zasshi*, Vol.122, No.5, pp.323-329, ISSN 0031-6903

Paine, MF., Criss, AB. and Watkins, PB. (2004). Two major grapefruit juice components differ in intestinal CYP3A4 inhibition kinetic and binding properties. *Drug Metab Dispos*, Vol.32, No.10, pp.1146-1153,

Rashid, J., McKinstry, C., Renwick, AG., Dirnhuber, M., Waller, DG. and George, CF. (1993). Quercetin, an in vitro inhibitor of CYP3A, does not contribute to the interaction between nifedipine and grapefruit juice. *Br J Clin Pharmacol*, Vol.36, No.5, pp.460-463,

Rashid, TJ., Martin, U., Clarke, H., Waller, DG., Renwick, AG. and George, CF. (1995). Factors affecting the absolute bioavailability of nifedipine. *Br J Clin Pharmacol*, Vol.40, No.1, pp.51-58,

Row, EC., Brown, SA., Stachulski, AV. and Lennard, MS. (2006). Design, synthesis and evaluation of furanocoumarin monomers as inhibitors of CYP3A4. *Org Biomol Chem*, Vol.4, No.8, pp.1604-1610,

Rush, WR., Alexander, O., Hall, DJ., Cairncross, L., Dow, RJ. and Graham, DJ. (1986). The metabolism of nicardipine hydrochloride in healthy male volunteers. *Xenobiotica*, Vol.16, No.4, pp.341-349, ISSN 0049-8254

Saita, T., Fujito, H. and Mori, M. (2004). Screening of furanocoumarin derivatives in citrus fruits by enzyme-linked immunosorbent assay. *Biol Pharm Bull*, Vol.27, No.7, pp.974-977, ISSN 0918-6158

Schmiedlin-Ren, P., Edwards, DJ., Fitzsimmons, ME., He, K., Lown, KS., Woster, PM., Rahman, A., Thummel, KE., Fisher, JM., Hollenberg, PF. and Watkins, PB. (1997). Mechanisms of enhanced oral availability of CYP3A4 substrates by grapefruit constituents. Decreased enterocyte CYP3A4 concentration and mechanism-based inactivation by furanocoumarins. *Drug Metab Dispos*, Vol.25, No.11, pp.1228-1233,

Schwarz, UI., Seemann, D., Oertel, R., Miehlke, S., Kuhlisch, E., Fromm, MF., Kim, RB., Bailey, DG. and Kirch, W. (2005). Grapefruit juice ingestion significantly reduces talinolol bioavailability. *Clin Pharmacol Ther*, Vol.77, No.4, pp.291-301,

Sigusch, H., Hippius, M., Henschel, L., Kaufmann, K. and Hoffmann, A. (1994). Influence of grapefruit juice on the pharmacokinetics of a slow release nifedipine formulation. *Pharmazie*, Vol.49, No.7, pp.522-524, ISSN 0031-7144

Soons, PA., Vogels, BA., Roosemalen, MC., Schoemaker, HC., Uchida, E., Edgar, B., Lundahl, J., Cohen, AF. and Breimer, DD. (1991). Grapefruit juice and cimetidine inhibit stereoselective metabolism of nitrendipine in humans. *Clin Pharmacol Ther*, Vol.50, No.4, pp.394-403, ISSN 0009-9236

Spahn-Langguth, H. and Langguth, P. (2001). Grapefruit juice enhances intestinal absorption of the P-glycoprotein substrate talinolol. *Eur J Pharm Sci*, Vol.12, No.4, pp.361-367, ISSN 0928-0987

Sugawara, K. (1996). Optimal use for drugs. *Pharm Mon*, Vol.38, pp.2591-2596, ISSN Pharm Mon

Takanaga, H., Ohnishi, A., Murakami, H., Matsuo, H., Higuchi, S., Urae, A., Irie, S., Furuie, H., Matsukuma, K., Kimura, M., Kawano, K., Orii, Y., Tanaka, T. and Sawada, Y. (2000). Relationship between time after intake of grapefruit juice and the effect on pharmacokinetics and pharmacodynamics of nisoldipine in healthy subjects. *Clin Pharmacol Ther*, Vol.67, No.3, pp.201-214,

Tassaneeyakul, W., Guo, LQ., Fukuda, K., Ohta, T. and Yamazoe, Y. (2000). Inhibition selectivity of grapefruit juice components on human cytochromes P450. *Arch Biochem Biophys*, Vol.378, No.2, pp.356-363,

Terashita, S., Tokuma, Y., Fujiwara, T., Shiokawa, Y., Okumura, K. and Noguchi, H. (1987). Metabolism of nilvadipine, a new dihydropyridine calcium antagonist, in rats and dogs. *Xenobiotica*, Vol.17, No.12, pp.1415-1425, ISSN 0049-8254

Tetko, IV. and Tanchuk, VY. (2002). Application of associative neural networks for prediction of lipophilicity in ALOGPS 2.1 program. *J Chem Inf Comput Sci*, Vol.42, No.5, pp.1136-1145, ISSN 0095-2338

Uesawa, Y., Abe, M., Fukuda, E., Baba, M., Okada, Y. and Mohri, K. (2011a). Construction of a model to estimate the CYP3A inhibitory effect of grapefruit juice. *Pharmazie*, Vol.66, No.7, pp.525-528, ISSN 0031-7144

Uesawa, Y., Abe, M. and Mohri, K. (2008). White and colored grapefruit juice produce similar pharmacokinetic interactions. *Pharmazie*, Vol.63, No.8, pp.598-600, ISSN 0031-7144

Uesawa, Y. and Mohri, K. (2005). Comprehensive determination of furanocoumarin derivatives in citrus juice by high performance liquid chromatography. *Yakugaku Zasshi*, Vol.125, No.11, pp.875-879, ISSN 0031-6903

Uesawa, Y. and Mohri, K. (2006). The use of heat treatment to eliminate drug interactions due to grapefruit juice. *Biol Pharm Bull*, Vol.29, No.11, pp.2274-2278, ISSN 0918-6158

Uesawa, Y. and Mohri, K. (2008a). Hesperidin in orange juice reduces the absorption of celiprolol in rats. *Biopharm Drug Dispos*, Vol.29, No.3, pp.185-188, ISSN 0142-2782

Uesawa, Y. and Mohri, K. (2008b). Drug interaction potentials among different brands of grapefruit juice. *Pharmazie*, Vol.63, No.2, pp.144-146, ISSN 0031-7144

Uesawa, Y. and Mohri, K. (2008c). Relationship between lipophilicities of 1,4-dihydropyridine derivatives and pharmacokinetic interaction strengths with grapefruit juice. *Yakugaku Zasshi*, Vol.128, No.1, pp.117-122, ISSN 0031-6903

Uesawa, Y. and Mohri, K. (2010). Quantitative structure-activity relationship (QSAR) analysis of the inhibitory effects of furanocoumarin derivatives on cytochrome P450 3A activities. *Pharmazie*, Vol.65, No.1, pp.41-46, ISSN 0031-7144

Uesawa, Y., Takeuchi, T. and Mohri, K. (2011b). *Curr Pharm Biotechnol*,.ISSN 1389-2010 (in press)

Uno, T., Ohkubo, T., Motomura, S. and Sugawara, K. (2006). Effect of grapefruit juice on the disposition of manidipine enantiomers in healthy subjects. *Br J Clin Pharmacol*, Vol.61, No.5, pp.533-537,

Uno, T., Ohkubo, T., Sugawara, K., Higashiyama, A., Motomura, S. and Ishizaki, T. (2000). Effects of grapefruit juice on the stereoselective disposition of nicardipine in humans: evidence for dominant presystemic elimination at the gut site. *Eur J Clin Pharmacol*, Vol.56, No.9-10, pp.643-649, ISSN 0031-6970

Vincent, J., Harris, SI., Foulds, G., Dogolo, LC., Willavize, S. and Friedman, HL. (2000). Lack of effect of grapefruit juice on the pharmacokinetics and pharmacodynamics of amlodipine. *Br J Clin Pharmacol*, Vol.50, No.5, pp.455-463,

Wang, R., Fu, Y. and Lai, L. (1997). A New Atom-Additive Method for Calculating Partition Coefficients. *J Chem Inf Comput Sci*, Vol.37, No.3, pp.615-621, ISSN 0095-2338

Watanabe, J. and Kozaki, A. (1978). Relationship between partition coefficients and apparent volumes of distribution for basic drugs. II. *Chem Pharm Bull (Tokyo)*, Vol.26, No.11, pp.3463-3470, ISSN 0009-2363

Yajima, Y., Iijima, H. and Yokoyama, R. (2003). Influence of grapefruit juice on the plasma concentration of efonidipine hydrochloride (Landel). *Yakuri To Chiryo*, Vol.31, No.7, pp.579-588, ISSN Yakuri To Chiryo

Yamada, Y., Ito, K., Nakamura, K., Sawada, Y. and Iga, T. (1993). Prediction of therapeutic doses of beta-adrenergic receptor blocking agents based on quantitative structure-pharmacokinetic/pharmacodynamic relationship. *Biol Pharm Bull*, Vol.16, No.12, pp.1251-1259, ISSN 0918-6158

Yamazaki, K. and Kanaoka, M. (2004). Computational prediction of the plasma protein-binding percent of diverse pharmaceutical compounds. *J Pharm Sci*, Vol.93, No.6, pp.1480-1494, ISSN 0022-3549

Zaidenstein, R., Soback, S., Gips, M., Avni, B., Dishi, V., Weissgarten, Y., Golik, A. and Scapa, E. (2001). Effect of grapefruit juice on the pharmacokinetics of losartan and its active metabolite E3174 in healthy volunteers. *Ther Drug Monit*, Vol.23, No.4, pp.369-373, ISSN 0163-4356

7

Drug Interaction Exposures in an Intensive Care Unit: Population Under Antihypertensive Use

Érica Freire de Vasconcelos-Pereira[1],
Mônica Cristina Toffoli-Kadri[1,*], Leandro dos Santos Maciel Cardinal[2]
and Vanessa Terezinha Gubert de Matos[3]
[1]Center of Biological and Health Sciences, Federal University of Mato Grosso do Sul,
[2]Multiprofessional Health Residence – Critical Care Patient,
[3]Section of Hospital Pharmacy, University Medical Centre,
Federal University of Mato Grosso do Sul,
Brazil

1. Introduction

A potential drug-drug interaction (DDI) is related to the possibility of a drug to alter the effect of another drug simultaneously administered. It can occur before or after drug administration (Almeida et al., 2007). DDI are considered predictable and thus avoidable and manageable (Cruciol-Souza et al., 2006).

Many of these interactions have slow onset clinical manifestations that can be diagnosed as new diseases and handled wrongly (Correr et al., 2007). Drug interactions are estimated to occur between 3% and 5% in patients to whom few drugs are prescribed and 20% among those who use 10 to 20 drugs simultaneously (Ferreira Sobrinho et al., 2006). The incidence of drug interactions is directly proportional to the increase in the number of drugs prescribed (Matos et al., 2009). It is known that a prescription containing eight or more drugs will present at least one interaction (Almeida et al., 2007).

Drug interactions incidence in Intensive Care Unit (ICU) is higher than hospital rates in general probably due to patient disease severity admitted in this unit (Almeida et al., 2007). ICU patients usually need great number of administered drugs and they are under risk of 44.3% to 95.0% of potential drug interactions occurrence (Sierra et al., 1997; Meneses & Monteiro, 2000). New drugs availability and prescription of fixed drug combinations difficult potential interactions identification (Trato, 2005). Thereby, this study aimed to discuss the risk of DDI in medical prescriptions of adult inpatients in ICU under use of antihypertensive drugs.

Commonly used drugs in ICU are vasoconstrictors and cardiotonic agents, antimicrobials, coronary vasodilators, direct vasodilators, antisecretory drugs, anticoagulants, sedatives-

---

[*] Corresponding Author

hypnotics agents, antiemetics, antidiabetics agents, analgesics-antipyretics and antiinflammatory drugs.

Micromedex® DrugReax® System (Klasco, 2011) is one of the most used database to describe interactions. The DrugReax System contains a dictionary of more than 8,000 unique drug terms. This system distinguishes trade names from equivalent generic names and it analyses specific drug instead of drug class. This database provides information about clinical consequences or adverse drug reactions that could result from a DDI, describe the interaction mechanism and classifies onset, severity and scientific knowledge of adverse reactions caused by the DDI.

Onset is classified as rapid (effects expected within 24 hours of drug administration), delayed (effects not expected to appear within the first 24 hours following drug administration) or unknown (effects expected to appear any time after drug administration).

Severity is classified as minor (limited clinical effects including increased frequency or severity of adverse effects and generally no major alteration in therapy), moderate (exacerbation of patient's condition and/or an alteration in therapy), major (life-threatening interaction and/or medical intervention to minimize or prevent serious adverse effects) or contraindicated (life-threatening interaction).

Scientific knowledge is classified considering how well DDI is documented in the literature that means excellent (controlled studies clearly established the existence of the interaction), good (documentation strongly suggests the interaction exists but well-controlled studies are lacking), fair (available documentation is poor but pharmacologic considerations lead clinicians to suspect about interaction existence or documentation is good for a pharmacologically similar drug) or unknown (no documentation about the interaction).

Table 1 presents the classification of DDI involving antihypertensive and the most frequent used drugs in ICU.

Antihypertensives	Drug Classes	Severity	Onset	Scientific knowledge	DDI Outcome
Calcium channel blockers	Histamine H2-antagonists (cimetidine)	Moderate	Rapid	Good	Increased concentrations of calcium channel blockers and possible cardiovascular toxicity
	Benzodiazepinics	Moderate	Rapid	Good	Increased/prolonged sedation
	Opioid analgesics	Major	Rapid	Good	Severe hypotension and an increased risk of respiratory depression
	Antifungals	Moderate	Delayed	Good	Increased calcium channel blockers concentrations and toxicity (dizziness, hypotension, flushing, headache, peripheral edema).

Antihypertensives	Drug Classes	Severity	Onset	Scientific knowledge	DDI Outcome
	Glucocorticoids	Moderate	Rapid	Good	Increased glucocorticoids concentrations and enhanced adrenal-suppressant effects
	Calcium channel blockers	Moderate	Rapid	Good	Toxicity (headache, peripheral edema, hypotension, tachycardia)
	Beta-blocker drugs	Major	Rapid	Good	Increased risk of hypotension, bradycardia, atrioventricular conduction disturbances
	Alpha 1-adrenergic blockers	Moderate	Rapid	Fair	Hypotension
	Alpha 2-adrenergic agonistic drug	Major	Not specified	Good	Increased incidence of sinus bradycardia requiring hospitalization and insertion of a pacemaker
Beta-blockers	Calcium channel blockers	Moderate	Rapid	Good	Hypotension and/or bradycardia
	Sympathomimetics	Major	Rapid	Excellent	Hypertension, bradycardia and resistance to epinephrine in anaphylaxis
	Hypoglycemic	Moderate	Delayed	Good	Hypoglycemia, hyperglycemia or hypertension
	Alpha 1-adrenergic blockers	Moderate	Rapid	Good	Exaggerated hypotensive response to the first dose of the alpha blocker
	Direct vasodilators	Moderate	Delayed	Fair	Increased risk of propranolol adverse effects (bradycardia, fatigue, bronchospasm)
	Lopp diuretics	Moderate	Rapid	Fair	Hypotension, bradycardia
	Thiazide diuretics	Moderate	Delayed	Fair	Hyperglycemia, hypertriglyceridemia
	Fluoroquinolone	Minor	Delayed	Fair	Bradycardia, hypotension
Lopp diuretics	Nonsteroidal antiinflammatory agents	Moderate	Delayed	Good	Decreased diuretic and antihypertensive efficacy
	Beta-blocker drugs	Moderate	Rapid	Fair	Hypotension, bradycardia
	Glucocorticoids	Moderate	Delayed	Fair	Hypokalemia

Antihypertensives	Drug Classes	Severity	Onset	Scientific knowledge	DDI Outcome
	Direct vasodilators	Minor	Rapid	Good	Enhanced diuretic response to loop diuretic
Potassium-sparing diuretics	Nonsteroidal antiinflammatory agents	Moderate	Delayed	Good	Reduced diuretic effectiveness, hyperkalemia, or possible nephrotoxicity
	Angiotensin converting enzyme inhibitors	Moderate	Delayed	Good	Hyperkalemia
	Angiotensin II Receptor Blockers	Moderate	Delayed	Fair	Hyperkalemia
Thiazide diuretics	Glucocorticoids	Moderate	Delayed	Fair	Hypokalemia and subsequent cardiac arrhythmias
	Nonsteroidal antiinflammatory agents	Moderate	Delayed	Good	Decreased diuretic and antihypertensive efficacy
	Beta-blockers	Moderate	Delayed	Fair	Hyperglycemia, hypertriglyceridemia
Angiotensin converting enzyme inhibitors	Nonsteroidal antiinflammatory agents	Moderate	Not specified	Excellent	Decreased antihypertensive efficacy
	Lopp diuretics	Moderate	Rapid	Good	Postural hypotension (first dose)
	Thiazide diuretics	Moderate	Rapid	Good	Postural hypotension (first dose)
Catecholamine synthesis or release blockers	Beta-blockers	Moderate	Rapid	Fair	Exaggerated hypertensive response, tachycardia, or arrhythmias during physiologic stress or exposure to exogenous catecholamines
	Oxazolidinone	Contraindicated	Rapid	Good	Hypertensive crisis (headache, palpitation, neck stiffness)
Direct vasodilators	Lopp diuretics	Minor	Rapid	Good	Enhanced diuretic response to loop diuretic
Alpha 2-adrenergic blockers	Beta-blockers	Major	Not specified	Fair	Increased risk of sinus bradycardia; exaggerated clonidine withdrawal response (acute hypertension)

Table 1. Classification of DDI involving antihypertensive drugs in medical prescriptions of adult inpatients in ICU

2. DDI of major severity

The combination of calcium channel blockers with opioid analgesics is classified as major severity because it may result in severe hypotension and an increased risk of respiratory depression caused by fentanyl toxicity. For example, diltiazem is a moderate CYP3A4 inhibitor and fentanyl is a CYP3A4 substrate. The concurrent use may result in increased fentanyl plasma levels and fatal respiratory depression. Caution is necessary if these agents are given concurrently and use the lowest possible fentanyl dose. Patient should be carefully monitored for an extended period of time for fentanyl adverse events. Any dosage increases to either medication should be made carefully.

Calcium channel blockers and beta-blocker drugs co-administration is also classified as major severity because it may result in an increased risk of hypotension, bradycardia, atrioventricular conduction disturbances. If concurrent therapy is required, cardiac function and blood pressure should be carefully monitored, particularly in patients predisposed to heart failure. A dosage adjustment for hepatically metabolized beta blockers may be required.

The combination of calcium channel blockers with alpha 2-adrenergic agonistic drug is classified as major severity because it may result in increased incidence of sinus bradycardia requiring hospitalization and insertion of a pacemaker. Therefore, heart rate should be monitored when clonidine and verapamil or diltiazem are given concurrently.

The abrupt discontinuation of vasodilators may lead to a hyper-adrenergic attack causing acute myocardial infarction, stroke and/or other complications due to rebound vasoconstriction. This effect is known as antihypertensive drugs withdrawal. The most commonly drugs involved in this effect are the beta-blockers, centrally acting agents, direct vasodilators and calcium channel blockers (Kirk & Johnson, 1995).

Concomitant use of beta-blockers and clonidine provide the rebound effect after abrupt withdrawal of therapy. Clonidine by an agonistic effect on presynaptic alpha-2 receptors decreases noradrenaline release from postganglionic sympathetic neurons. It is an excess of catecholamines in the synaptic clefts when the administration of clonidine is interrupted and this catecholamines are available for binding to the alpha and beta receptors. However, if the beta receptor, auxiliar in vasodilation, is blocked, the alpha effects are not counterbalanced. The result is vasoconstriction, rebound hypertension and risk of coronary and cerebral vasospasm. It is recommended that in patients who are on beta blockers and clonidine, the drug should be withdrawn gradually to avoid this adverse drug reaction. Moreover, the use of clonidine and beta-blocker raises the risk of sinus bradycardia (Goodman & Gilman, 2011).

The concurrent use of beta-blocker and sympathomimetic drugs should be avoided because it may result in hypertension, bradycardia and resistance to epinephrine in anaphylaxis. However, if concomitant therapy is necessary, patient should be carefully monitored for severe and prolonged hypertension. Glucagon has positive inotropic and chronotropic effects that are independent of adrenergic receptors. The use of this agent is of great importance in patients on beta blockers which are affected by an anaphylactic reaction. Glucagon increases cardiac output and coronary perfusion, decreasing myocardial hypoxia and a possible secondary cardiogenic shock (Lieberman, 1998).

Alpha 2-adrenergic blockers and beta-blockers may result in increased risk of sinus bradycardia; exaggerated clonidine withdrawal response (acute hypertension). Monitor heart rate when clonidine and atenolol are given concurrently. Patients to be withdrawn from clonidine who are concomitantly receiving a beta blocking agent, such as atenolol, should be withdrawn from the beta blocker several days before the gradual discontinuation of clonidine to avoid an excessive rise in blood pressure. In the case of a hypertensive crisis following discontinuation of clonidine, IV phentolamine or oral clonidine can be used to reverse the excessive rise in blood pressure. Patients to be withdrawn from clonidine who are concomitantly receiving a beta blocking agent should be monitored carefully for hypertension.

3. Catecholamine synthesis or release blockers and oxazolidinone

The severity of the most frequent used drugs in ICU is moderate to minor. However, the combination of catecholamine synthesis or release blockers with oxazolidinone is contraindicated because it may result in hypertensive crisis, causing headache, palpitation and neck stiffness. Hypertension due to drugs can cause increase of blood pressure level, reduction of antihypertensive drug effectiveness or the worsening of a pre-existing hypertension.

Linezolida is an antibiotic used to treat infections caused by gram-positive bacteria but this drug is also a non-selective and reversible inhibitor of monoamine oxidase (MAO). The inhibitors of this enzyme block the oxidative deamination of three biogenic amines which are norepinephrine, dopamine and 5-hydroxytryptamine. When monoamine oxidase inhibitors (MAOI) are associated with sympathomimetic drugs or foods containing tyramine, hypertensive crisis may occur (Fuzikawa et al., 1999). The hypertensive crises are life-threatening and can also cause damage to susceptible organs as heart, brain and kidneys (Plavnik, 2002).

4. Calcium channel blockers and histamine H2-antagonists

The co-administration of calcium channel blockers and some histamine H2-antagonists, as cimetidine, result in increased concentrations of calcium channel blockers and possible cardiovascular toxicity. This effect happens because of Cytochrome P (CYP) 450 inhibition.

The Cytochrome P (CYP) 450 is a superfamily of hemoproteins that play an important role in the metabolism of steroid hormones, fatty acids and many drugs. Many agents used for management of cardiovascular diseases are substrates, inhibitors or inducers of CYP450 enzymes. When two agents that are substrates, inhibitors or inducers of CYP450 are administered together, drug interactions with significant clinical consequences may occur (Cheng et al., 2009). Monitoring cardiovascular response is necessary when the patient is in use of cimetidine and a calcium channel blocker. Dose reductions of up to 35% to 40% may be needed for diltiazem or nifedipine if co-administered with cimetidine.

5. Antihypertensive and antiinflammatory agents

5.1 Nonsteroidal antiinflammatory agents

Nonsteroidal antiinflammatory drugs (NSAID) may block the antihypertensive effects of thiazide and loop diuretics, β-adrenergic blockers, α-adrenergic blockers and angiotensin-converting enzyme inhibitors. It seems to happen by NSAID interference with prostaglandins synthesis which may thus limit the ability of antihypertensive drugs to control blood pressure.

When concomitant use of loop diuretics and NSAID is required, patient should be monitored for diuretic efficacy and for signs of renal failure.

Potassium-sparing diuretics and NSAID co-administration may also result in hyperkalemia or possible nephrotoxicity. If this combination is necessary, patient should be monitored for blood pressure, weight changes, urine output, potassium levels, creatinine levels, decreased effectiveness of the diuretic and hyperkalemia.

In same way, when concurrently administration of thiazide diuretics and NSAID is necessary, blood pressure and weight should be monitored. It is important to follow the patient for signs of renal failure, including decreases in urine output and increased edema.

Caution is recommended when prescribing NSAID to patients taking ACE inhibitors. When concomitant use is required, patient should be monitored for ACE inhibitor efficacy and for signs of renal failure. NSAID may also promote the development of hyperkalemia in association with ACE inhibitors as a result of deterioration of renal function. They are also responsible for reducing the antihypertensive effects of ACEI by interfering in the synthesis of prostaglandins. Probenicid reduces captopril renal excretion and increases its plasma concentration. On the other hand, aspirin and antiacids may decrease or abolish the antihypertensive efficacy of captopril (Gonzaga et al., 2009).

The mechanism of the hypertensive effects caused by NSAID seems primarily to be related to their ability to block the cyclo-oxygenase pathway of arachidonic acid metabolism which results in decrease of prostaglandin formation. The prostaglandins are important in normal modulation of renal and systemic vascular dilatation, glomerular filtration, tubular secretion of salt and water reabsorption, adrenergic neurotransmission and the renin-angiotensin-aldosterone system. Blockade of benef3ic effects of prostaglandins by NSAID results in complexes events which culminate in attenuation of many antihypertensive agents effects. The risk is greatest in the elderly, blacks and patients with low-renin hypertension. (Houston, 1991).

Pharmacologically, it is thought that NSAID interact differently with antihypertensive drugs. However, the NSAID effects on newly initiated antihypertensive drug therapy remain unclear because few studies have included patients who were initially administered NSAID and then antihypertensives. Physiologically, the effects of renal prostaglandins on salt and water transport in the kidney are complementary to the actions of diuretics. Therefore, it is likely that the blocking of prostaglandins synthesis by NSAID attenuates the effect of diuretics. angiotensin-converting enzyme (ACE) inhibitors produce vasodilatation and lower blood pressure by inhibiting ACE which promotes the formation of angiotensin-2 and aldosterone. Bradykinin is an autacoid that produces vasodilatation and further reduces blood pressure. Blocking ACE decreases the inhibition of bradykinin-induced vasodilatation. However, the vasodilatory properties of bradykinin that contribute to the antihypertensive properties of ACE inhibition appear to be mediated through local release of prostaglandins and are therefore susceptible to interference by NSAID (Ishiguro et al., 2008).

5.2 Steroidal antiinflammatory agents

Glucocorticoids may increase blood pressure by increasing the concentration of sodium-potassium adenosine triphosphate in the cell membrane which could increase the concentration of extracellular sodium and therefore expand the plasma volume. Cortisol also stimulates the synthesis of mineralocorticoid aldosterone leading to sodium and water retention and, consequently, increased blood volume and cardiac output (Ortega et al., 1996; Brown, 2005). It also increases the sensitivity of the myocardium to endogenous catecholamine and increases the vascular response to endogenous vasopressors such as angiotensin II and norepinephrine (Ortega et al., 1996). In addition, glucocorticoids induce hepatic production of angiotensinogen resulting in an exacerbated response of the renin-angiotensin-aldosterone system (Dukes, 1992).

6. Beta-blockers and hypoglycemic drugs

The use of beta-blockers and hypoglycemic may result in hypoglycemia, hyperglycemia or hypertension. If the use of a beta blocker is required in a diabetic patient, glucose should be carefully monitored. Cardioselective beta blockers (atenolol, metoprolol) cause less disturbance of glucose metabolism and less masking of hypoglycemic effects. Propranolol accounts for the majority of positive reports of interactions and should clearly be avoided.

Hyperglycemia occurs frequently in critically ill patients and it is a marker of poor prognosis (Pitrowsky et al., 2009). The main complication of insulin therapy is hypoglycemia which is considered a potentially serious adverse event in these patients (Diener et al., 2006). The combination of a beta-blocker and insulin may impose a higher risk of blood glucose changes and lead to the development of hypoglycemia, hyperglycemia and hypertension.

Beta-blockers may inhibit some of the normal physiologic response to hypoglycemia. Symptoms of hypoglycemia such as tremors and tachycardia may be absent, making it more difficult for patients to recognize an oncoming episode. In addition, multiple effects on glucose metabolism have been reported, usually with the noncardioselective beta-blockers (e.g., propranolol, pindolol, timolol) but occasionally also with relatively beta-1 selective agents (e.g., metoprolol). Specifically, inhibition of catecholamine-mediated glycogenolysis and glucose mobilization in association with beta-blockade can potentiate insulin-induced hypoglycemia in diabetics and delay the recovery of normal blood glucose levels. Prolonged and severe hypoglycemia may occur, although these events have rarely been reported. Significant increases in blood pressure and bradycardia can also occur during hypoglycemia in diabetics treated with insulin and beta-blockers due to antagonism of epinephrine's effect on beta-2 adrenergic receptors, which leads to unopposed alpha-adrenergic effects including vasoconstriction. Other effects reported with various beta-blockers include decreased glucose tolerance and decreased glucose-induced insulin secretion (Goodman & Gilman, 2010).

7. Conclusion

The need of multiple drugs simultaneously used is common in the intensive care environment and contribute to the occurrence of drug interactions. The clinical consequences of these interactions should be considered in order not to endanger ICU inpatients health once this population is under unfavorable conditions.

The presence of drug interactions is a permanent risk in the ICU and not all DDI can be prevented. The use of software is mentioned in the literature as an important toll in reviewing prescriptions to identify interactions and reduce adverse events. Also, the continuing education of professionals involved in the processes of prescribing, dispensing and administering medicines as the main risk factors for drug interactions, the dissemination of information regarding the more frequent and important in clinical practice about drug interactions are instruments in the prevention of drug interactions.

8. References

[1] AHFS Drug Information 2006. American Society of Health-System Pharmacists. Editor Gerald K. McEvoy. Bethseda, Maryland - USA, 3776p.
Gerald K. McEvoy, American Society of Health-System Pharmacists.(2006). *AHFS Drug Information*. Bethseda, ISBN 1585281425, Maryland - USA.

[2] Almeida, SM; Gama, CS & Akamine, N. (2007). Prevalência e classificação de interações entre medicamentos dispensados para pacientes em terapia intensiva. *Einstein*, v. 5, n. 4, p. 347-351, ISSN 1679-4508.

[3] Brown, S.A. (2005) Pathophysiology of systemic hypertension. In: ETTINGER, S.; FELDMAN, E.C. (Ed.6), Textbook of Veterinary Internal Medicine. Missouri: Elsevier Saunders, Cap.29, p. 472-476.
Brown, S.A. (2005). Pathophysiology of systemic hypertension. In: *Textbook of Veterinary Internal Medicine*. Ettinger, S.; Feldman, p. 472-476, ISBN 1-4160-0110-7, Missouri: Elsevier Saunders.

[4] Cheng, JWM; Frishman, W & Aronow, WS. (2009). Updates on Cytochrome P450-Mediated Cardiovascular Drug Interactions. *American Journal of Therapeutics*.v.16 n.2, p.155-163, ISSN 1075-2765.

[5] Correr, CJ; Pontarolo, R; Ferreira, LC & Baptistão, SAM. (2007). Riscos de problemas relacionados com medicamentos em pacientes de uma instituição geriátrica. *Revista Brasileira Ciências Farmacêutica*.v.43,n.1,p.55-62, ISSN 1516-9332.

[6] Cruciol-Souza, JM; Thomson ,JC & Catisti, DG. (2008). Avaliação de prescrições medicamentosas de um hospital universitário brasileiro. *Revista brasileira educação médica*.v. 32, n.2, p.188–196, ISSN 0100-5502.

[7] Diener, JRC; Prazeres, CEE; Rosa, CM; Alberton, UC & Ramos, CCS. (2006). Avaliação da Efetividade e Segurança do Protocolo de Infusão de Insulina de Yale para o Controle Glicêmico Intensivo. *Revista Brasileira Terapia Intensiva*. v.18, n.3, p.268-275, ISSN 0103-507X.

[8] Dukes, J. (1992).Hypertension: A review of the mechanisms, manifestations and management. *Journal of Small Animal Practice*, v.33, n.3, p.119-129, ISSN 00224510.

[9] Ferreira Sobrinho, F; Nascimento, JWL; Greco, KV & Menezes FG. (2006). Avaliação de interações medicamentosas em prescrições de pacientes hospitalizados. *Revista Racine*.v.16, n.94, p.67-70, ISSN 1807-166X.

[10] Fuzikawa, CS; Hara, C; Glória, MBA & Rocha, FL. (1999). IMAO e Dieta: Atualização - orientações práticas para o uso clínico. *Jornal Brasileiro Psiquiatria*. v.48, n.10, p.453-60, ISSN 0047-2085.

[11] Gonzaga, CC; Passarelli Jr., O & Amodeo, C. (2009). Drugs interactions: angiotensin-converting enzyme inhibitors, angiotensin II-receptor antagonists, renin inhibitors. *Revista Brasileira Hipertensão*. v.16, n.4, p.221-225, ISSN 1519-7522.

[12] Goodman, L.S & A. Gilman. (2010) As bases farmacológicas da terapêutica. 11 ed. LLBruntan; JS Lazo;KL Parker. McGrawl-hill, Rio de Janeiro: Guanabara Koogan. Goodman, LS & Gilman, A. (11 ed). (2010). *As bases farmacológicas da terapêutica*.McGrawl-hill, ISBN 85-7726-001-1, Rio de Janeiro.

[13] Houston, MC. (1991) Nonsteroidal anti-inflammatory drugs and antihypertensives. The American Journal of *Medicine*. v. 90 n.5, Suppl. 1, p. S42-47, *ISSN 0002-9343*.

[14] Ishiguro, C; Fujita, T; Omori, T; Fujii, Y; Mayama, T & Sato, T. (2008).Assessing the Effects of Non-steroidal Anti-inflammatory Drugs on Antihypertensive Drug Therapy Using Post-Marketing Surveillance Database. *Journal of Epidemiology*. v.18, n.3,p. 119-124, ISSN 1349-9092 .

[15] Klasco RK (editor): DRUG-REAX® System. Thomson MICROMEDEX, Greenwood Village, Colorado. Accessed in Oct 2011.

[16] Kirk JK & Johnson SH. (1995). Safe Discontinuation of Antihypertensive Therapy. *Archives Family Medicine*. v. n.4, p.266-270, ISSN 1063-3987.

[17] Lieberman, P. (1998) Anaphylaxis and Anaphylactoid Reactions. In: *Allergy – principles and pratice* Middleton E; Ellis EF; Reed CE; Adkinson NF; Yunginger JW & Busse WW, eds., 5 ed, Mosby, Saint Louis.

[18] Mark, CH. (1991).Nonsteroidal anti-inflammatory drugs and antihypertensives. *The American Journal of Medicine*, v. 90 n.5, Suppl. 1, p. S42-47, ISSN 0002-9343.

[19] Matos, VTG; Vasconcelos, EF; Amaral, MS & Toffoli-Kadri, MC. (2009). Avaliação das Interações Medicamentosas em Prescrições Hospitalares de Pacientes Sob Uso de Anti-Hipertensivos. *Latin American Journal of Pharmacy*. v. 28, n. 4, p. 501-6, ISSN: 0326-2383.

[20] Meneses, A; Monteiro HS. (2000). Prevalência de interações medicamentosas "droga-droga" potenciais em duas UTIs (pública X privada) de Fortaleza, Brasil. *Revista Brasileira Terapia Intensiva*.v. 12, n.1, p.4-7, ISSN 0103-507X.

[21] Ortega, TM; Feldman, EC; Nelson, RW; Willits, N & Cowgill, LD. (1996) Sistemic arterial blood pressure and urine protein/creatinine ratio in dogs with hyperadrenocorticism. *Journal* of the *American Veterinary Medical Association*, v. 209, n. 10, p.1724-1729, ISSN 0003-1488.

[22] Plavnik, FL. (2002).Hipertensão arterial induzida por drogas: como detectar e tratar. *Revista Brasileira Hipertensão*. v. 9, n.2, p. 185-191, ISSN *1519-7522*.

[23] Pitrowsky, M; Shinotsuka CR; Soares M & Salluh JIF. (2009). Controle glicêmico em terapia intensiva 2009: sem sustos e sem surpresas. *Revista Brasileira Terapia Intensiva*. v.21, n.3, p. 310-314, ISSN 0103-507*X*.

[24] Sierra, P; Castillo, J; Gómez, M; Sorribes, V; Monterde, J & Castaño J. (1997). Potential and real drug interactions in critical care patients. *Revista Española Anestesiologia y Reanimación*. v. 44, n.10 p.383-7, ISSN *0034-9356*.

[25] Trato, DS. (2005). *Drug interactions facts*. St Louis: Facts and Comparisons. ISBN 157439195X

8

The Use of Antihypertensive Medicines in Primary Health Care Settings

Marc Twagirumukiza[1,2], Jan De Maeseneer[2], Thierry Christiaens[1,2], Robert Vander Stichele[1] and Luc Van Bortel[1]
[1]*Heymans Institute of Pharmacology, Ghent University, Ghent,*
[2]*Department of Family Medicine and Primary Health Care, Ghent University, Ghent, Belgium*

1. Introduction

This chapter is drawing out the patterns and evidences for the use of antihypertensive medicines in general and in primary health care settings in particular. It presents the overview of the recent advances in clinical effectiveness of the antihypertensive medicines, but also document the implication for management of hypertension in low level health facilities. The discussions are based on the new evidences from clinical practice, reviews and meta-analysis studies.

The chapter as whole is written from a comprehensive health care system development rather than from a purely medicines description perspective. Finally the authors do not intend to substitute the students or prescribers vademecum or medicines' handbooks but providing an update in their daily questions when comes the issue of whom, what (and with what) to treat – as far as arterial hypertension is concerned, in primary health care settings.

2. Rationale, objectives and methods

Hypertension, also known as "high blood pressure" is currently the major risk factor for coronary heart disease (Roger VL. and others 2011) and cerebrovascular disease (stroke) (Roger VL. and others 2011; Twagirumukiza and others 2011). Already known as significant public health problem worldwide particularly in western societies (Kearney and others 2005), hypertension has been documented recently as real health threat in developing countries as well (Kearney and others 2005; Twagirumukiza and others 2011). Hypertension remains the leading reason for office visits in primary care (Pittrow and others 2004) in some western countries in contrast with developing countries where awareness is still low and where hypertensive patients reach health facilities rather for complications. This situation in developing countries, emphasizes the need of other approaches and strategies to avert the Non Communicable Diseases (NCDs) in general and the arterial hypertension morbidity and mortality in particular by targeting the lower level of the health system chain (De Maeseneer J. and others 2011).

On the other side, despite the availability of a wide range of antihypertensive drugs (Van Bortel and others 2011), blood pressure has remained poorly controlled in a majority of health care settings, particularly in low resource settings. The access to medicines is highly driven by the availability and the cost of these drugs and strongly influences the prescription and usage patterns which in the end affect control of blood pressure(Twagirumukiza and others 2010). The rational use of available resources and the integration of the management strategies at primary health care level (De Maeseneer J 2009) have been advocated as key point of improving hypertension treatment (Twagirumukiza and Van Bortel 2011).

The aim of this chapter summarize the current knowledge on the use of antihypertensives in primary care and to provide an update to prescribers and health professionals in their daily questions about whom-and-how to treat -as far as arterial hypertension is concerned.

3. Epidemiology of hypertension

Arterial hypertension (HT) refers to a permanently and abnormally elevated arterial blood pressure . Arterial blood pressure (BP) corresponds to the force exerted by the circulating blood on the walls of blood vessels, and constitutes one of the cardinal vital clinical signs (Nichols WW. and others 2011). Hypertension can be classified either essential (primary) or secondary. Essential hypertension indicates that no specific medical cause can be found to explain a patient's condition. Secondary hypertension indicates that the high blood pressure is a result of (i.e., secondary to) another condition, such as kidney disease or tumours (pheochromocytoma among others). In current usage, the word "hypertension" once used without a qualifier will refers to essential systemic, arterial hypertension.

According to the World Health Organization (WHO) (World Health Organization and others 2004), hypertension is one of 7 diseases composing the entity of "cardiovascular diseases" (CVDs). This entity list includes, besides hypertension, coronary heart disease, cerebrovascular disease, peripheral artery disease, rheumatic heart disease, congenital heart disease and heart failure (Lopez and others 2006; World Health Organization and others 2004). By its target organ damage (TOD) hypertension remains an important cause of coronary heart disease, cerebrovascular disease, peripheral artery disease, and heart failure, which counts together with congenital heart disease for more than 75% of the CVDs morbi-mortality worldwide. The epidemiology of hypertension is therefore linked to CVDs and within this chapter, is considered both as a disease and as a risk factor for other CVDs.

Cardiovascular diseases, especially hypertension and related risk factors are of real health concern worldwide (Lawes and others 2008). Currently, the majority of hypertensive people live in developing regions (Kearney and others 2005), where their number is presumed to increase in coming decades (Kearney and others 2005), which inevitably will lead to a higher burden of cardiovascular diseases (Kearney and others 2005; Murray and Lopez 1997). Within a context of limited data on the burden of hypertension and other chronic diseases in many developing countries (Murray and Lopez 1997), those diseases are very often considered as uncommon and therefore they are rarely addressed by policy makers (Unwin and others 2001) who are very often focused on a well described predominance of infectious diseases in these regions (Unwin and others 2001).

Nevertheless, hypertension should be considered of great economic importance also in developing countries and regions like in Latina America, South Asia and sub-Saharan Africa, because it is frequently underdiagnosed, and frequently undertreated, as patients often cannot afford treatment. In such situations, the complications of hypertension are more frequent and more severe: mainly heart failure (Mensah 2003) and stroke (Mufunda J and others 2006). In addition if developing world inhabitants survive to adulthood, hypertension-related disease may be the major cause of premature mortality (Twagirumukiza and others 2009b). The prevalence of hypertension has been well described worldwide (Kearney and others 2005) and in sub-Saharan Africa (Twagirumukiza and others 2011). The current figures and their projections remain overwhelming. Currently around 972 million people have hypertension worldwide (rising up to 1.6 billion in 2025) and more than 65% of them are in developing countries (Kearney and others 2005). The 2008 number of hypertensives in sub-Saharan Africa is estimated at 74.7 million (increasing by 68.0% in 2025(Twagirumukiza and others 2011)).The prevalence of hypertension in this region is estimated at 16.2%, being higher in urban than in rural regions (Twagirumukiza and others 2011). This prevalence adjusted to WHO standard population is similar to the prevalence in western countries (Table 1).

Table 1 shows that although the prevalence of hypertension was lower in sub-Saharan Africa than in England and USA, the prevalence of hypertension adjusted to the WHO standard population was higher in sub-Saharan Africa than in England and tended to be higher than in USA. However, the analysis of age-specific prevalence data shows that the hypertension prevalence is higher at younger ages (up to 35 years) in sub-Saharan Africa compared to the western countries, indicating that hypertension starts at earlier age in sub-Saharan Africa. The prevalence in old people is lower in sub-Saharan Africa than in western country. The plausible explanation is linked to low accessibility to treatment: by lacking adequate treatment people with hypertension at younger age died in earlier ages (around 45-54 years). People with hypertension at older age are new cases or survivors.

There are evidences (Twagirumukiza and others 2011) of a clear difference in hypertension prevalence between countries. Different factors like diet habits (i.e. salt consumption) and genetic predisposition may play a role. As expected the prevalence of hypertension also increases with age and that prevalence was 50.7% higher in urban than in rural area. The influence of urbanization on hypertension was more pronounced in males than in females. These observations in rural versus urban areas are in line with other recent reports (Opie and Seedat 2005) reporting urban prevalence 1.5 to 2 times higher than rural ones. This difference can be influenced by the habits in rural which are dominated by routine field work as compared to urban lifestyle with more consumption of energy rich foods and a decrease in energy expenditure through less physical activity (Opie and Seedat 2005). However, modernisation (Dominguez and others 2006) may also transform rural settings themselves such as increasing use of automobiles leading to a decrease in physical activity, increasing overweight and obesity and more consumption of salt (Mufunda J and others 2006; Reddy and Yusuf 1998) and tobacco (Jha P and Chaloupka F 1999).

In sub-Saharan Africa setting, hypertension occurs earlier among adults of working age and its complications strike people at the top of their economic activity (Gaziano 2005; Twagirumukiza and others 2009b). Apart from the consequences on the quality of individual health, this leads to a large impact on a developing country's economic viability. In South Africa, for example, 2% to 3% of the country's gross national income, or roughly 25% of South African healthcare expenditures, was devoted to the direct treatment of cardiovascular disease (CVD) (Gaziano 2005; Pestana and others 1996).

	Crude hypertension prevalence in % (number of diagnosed hypertensive people/sample size)			Statistical comparison test p-value		
Age-range[a]	[1]sub-Saharan Africa	[2] England	[3] USA	Within all	sub-Saharan Africa vs England	sub-Saharan Africa vs USA
15-34	6.9 (19,366,486/281,419,841)	4.2 (33,461/798,390)	6.0 (178/2,971)	<0.001	<0.001*	<0.001*
35-44	17.1 (12,788,663/74,689,253)	12.3 (60,128/487,692)	16.0 (135/846)	<0.001	<0.001*	NS
45-54	28.8 (14,195,235/49,276,086)	26.3 (102,484/389,053)	31.0 (242/781)	<0.001	<0.001*	NS
55-64	44.0 (13,886,165/31,526,626)	45.8 (162,533/355,094)	48.0 (312/650)	0.045	0.004	NS
≥65	60.1 (14,470,484/24,074,117)	61.2 (333,947/545,786)	71.4 (849/1,189)	<0.001	NS	<0.001
Overall	16.2 (74,707,034/460,985,923)	26.9 (692,553/2,576,015)	26.7 (1,716/6,437)	<0.001	<0.001	<0.001
Prevalence standardized for WHO standard population **[4]**	22.3	18.4	21.6	<0.001	<0.001*	NS

[a] Age range for USA prevalence starts from 18 years, for England are from 16 years and for sub-Saharan Africa are from 15 years; **[1]** Results from a meta-analysis on the population-based studies(Twagirumukiza and others 2011); **[2]** Results from the Health Improvement Network (THIN) database & Health Survey for England (HSE)(MacDonald and Morant 2008); **[3]** NHANES III continuous(Fields and others 2004); **[4]** WHO standard population adjusted prevalence; **NS:** Not statistically significant *sub-Saharan Africa is statistically higher.

Table 1. Comparison between sub-Saharan Africa pooled data and developed countries surveys.

4. Management of hypertension in primary health care

4.1 Definitions challenges, and first drug choice

Up from what level a blood pressure is considered as high or as hypertension has been a constant discussion over time. Since the relationship between blood pressure and adverse health effects displays a non-linear but continuous relationship (John KJ Li 2000), any classification of people into dichotomous categories ('normotensive' and 'hypertensive') as well as other blood pressure staging are arbitrary (Mancia and others 2007). Nevertheless, clinicians and other health care workers often must make essentially dichotomous decisions (Birkett 1997) (e.g. whether or not to start pharmacological treatment for elevated blood pressure). The basis for classifying people into 'hypertensive' and 'normotensive' groups is encouraged by a consideration of 'excess risk' or by proven treatment benefit in clinical trials (Birkett 1997) for a certain level of blood pressure.

The definition of hypertension is then based on the potential of blood pressure to become a risk for cardiovascular events (Khosla and Black 2006). But this evaluation of potential risk has been improving in time and cut-offs have been lowered progressively. Previously, hypertension started at a cut-off SBP/DBP value of 160/95 mmHg, whereas the current standard is 140/90 mmHg. The current definition of hypertension which is unanimously agreed on by USA Joint National Committee on Detection, Evaluation, and Treatment of High Blood Pressure (JNC7)(Chobanian and others 2003), European Society of Hypertension (ESH) and of the European Society of Cardiology (ESC)(Mancia and others 2007) and World Health Organization (WHO)(Chalmers and others 1999) is : **SBP ≥ 140mmHg and/or DBP ≥ 90mmHg and/or being on blood pressure lowering medication**(Chalmers and others 1999; Chobanian and others 2003; Mancia and others 2007). These cut-off values are even lower in high risk population (diabetes or renal failure). Different thresholds have been given for different types of measurements (Table 2).

Situations	SBP	DBP
Office or clinic	140	90
Ambulatory 24-hour	125–130	80
Day	130–135	85
Night	120	70
Home	130–135	85

Table 2. Different Blood pressure thresholds (mmHg)(Mancia and others 2007)

In daily practice, the blood pressure has also been splitted up into grades to help management. In this chapter, the most recent (2007) classification (Mancia and others 2007) will be used as a reference.

SBP/DBP (mmHg)	WHO/ISH (2003)	JNC-7 (2003)	ESH/ESC (2007)
<120/80	-	Normal	Optimal
120-129/80-84	-	Pre-hypertension	Normal
130-139/85-89	-		High normal
140-159/90-99	Hypertension grade 1	Hypertension stage 1	Hypertension grade 1 (mild)
160-179/100-109	Hypertension grade 2	Hypertension stage 2	Hypertension grade 2 (moderate)
≥180/110	Hypertension grade 3		Hypertension grade 3 (severe)
** ≥140/<90	-	-	Isolated systolic hypertension

JNC-7: the Seventh report of the Joint National Committee on prevention, detection, evaluation, and treatment of high blood pressure (JNC-7)(Chobanian and others 2003). ESH/ESC: the European Society of Hypertension - European Society of Cardiology(Mancia and others 2007). WHO/ISH: the World Health Organization/ International Society of Hypertension(Whitworth 2003). Note that hypertension is defined as SBP/DBP of 140/90 mmHg according to the three recommendations(Chemla 2006).When a patient's systolic and diastolic blood pressure fall into different categories, the higher category should apply.

Table 3. Recent classifications and staging of Systolic (SBP) / Diastolic (DBP) Blood Pressure levels

In some patients, medical office blood pressure is persistently elevated while ambulatory or home blood pressure, are within their normal range. This condition is widely known as *'white coat hypertension'* (Mancia and others 2007). Inversely the hypertension found with ambulatory blood pressure measurement but not in clinic is known as *"masked hypertension"* (Papadopoulos and Makris 2007).

4.2 Cardiovascular risk evaluation

In aim to decide which drug to use, the patient risk needs to be evaluated. Many algorithms and charts have been released and some health professionals may be even confused. Authors argue that estimating risk is not the problem, but using it to tailor treatment to individuals is (Christiaens 2008). This section will not document all available charts in details , but will put forward the most useful risk assessment tool in the field.

Historically, hypertension guidelines focused on blood pressure values as the only or main variables determining the need and the type of treatment (Chobanian and others 2003). The current approach (Mancia and others 2007) emphasizes that diagnosis and management of hypertension should be related to quantification of total (or global) cardiovascular risk. List 1 shows those cardiovascular risk factors, including hypertension.

- **Risk factors that cannot be changed**
  - Age
  - Gender (male sex)
  - Family history of CV events and genetic predispositions (including ethnicity)
- **Risk factors that can be changed**
  - High blood pressure
  - Level of pulse pressure (in elderly)
  - Physical inactivity
  - Obesity and overweight
  - Smoking
  - Metabolic syndrome components:
    - Dyslipidaemia
      - High levels of total cholesterol level (TC)
      - High levels of Low density lipoprotein (LDL-c)
      - Elevated total triglycerides
    - Insulin resistance
    - Abnormal fasting plasma glucose
    - Abnormal glucose tolerance test
    - Abdominal obesity
    - Excessive alcohol consumption.
- **Other risk factors that can be managed**
  - Diabetes mellitus
  - Left ventricular hypertrophy
  - Chronic renal failure
  - Individual response to stress.
  - Plasma fibrinogen levels

List 1. List of cardiovascular(CV) risk factors(Mancia and others 2007)

It has been proposed (Mancia and others 2007) that the management of hypertension should be based on two criteria, i.e. (1) the level of systolic and diastolic blood pressure, and (2) the level of added cardiovascular risk (List 1). Thus, the management of hypertension has been shifted from viewing and treating it as an isolated element to a more comprehensive approach of cardiovascular risk stratification that takes into account other cardiovascular risk factors like cholesterol, smoking, diabetes and metabolic syndrome (MS). In addition, subclinical organ damage (List 2) is considered as higher added risk showing that risk factors led to organ damage.

The cardiovascular risk stratification table (Table 4) is obtained by combination of presence of risk factors, target organ damage and diabetes and the levels of systolic and diastolic blood pressure.

We have to keep in mind that many other risk tables have been developed as well. Hippisley-Cox and colleagues have developed and validated the second version of the QRISK cardiovascular disease risk algorithm (QRISK2), an attempt to more accurately estimate cardiovascular risk in patients from different ethnic groups in England and Wales(Christiaens 2008). The SCORE tables used the same risk factors to calculate corrected European cardiovascular mortality (Christiaens 2008). More recently the ASSIGN (Christiaens 2008) and now the QRISK tables (Christiaens 2008) tried to incorporate some other known risk factors, especially deprivation and family history.

All attempts to make risk tables more accurate, as done by Hippisley-Cox and colleagues in the QRISK2 algorithm (Christiaens 2008) should be welcomed. However, this is not the key problem. We have to fundamentally rethink how to use risk tables when making treatment decisions in practice, taking into consideration the prescribing in healthy older people and the correct use of drugs.

- Left Ventricular Hypertrophy (LVH):
  - Electrocardiographic LVH (Sokolow-Lyon >38 mm; Cornell >2440 mm*ms) or:
  - Echocardiographic LVH(LVMI M≥125 g/m2, W ≥110 g/m2)
- Carotid wall thickening (IMT > 0.9 mm) or plaque
- Carotid-femoral pulse wave velocity (PWV) >12 m/s
- Ankle/brachial BP index <0.9
- Slight increase in plasma creatinine:
  - Men (M): 115–133 μmol/l (1.3–1.5 mg/dl);
  - Women (W): 107–124 μmol/l (1.2–1.4 mg/dl)
- Low estimated glomerular filtration rate(<60 ml/min/1.73 m^2) or creatinine clearance (<60 ml/min)
- Microalbuminuria 30–300 mg/24 h or albumin-creatinine ratio: ≥22 (M) or ≥31 (W) mg/g creatinine

*Adapted from "2007 ESC/ESH Recommendations" (Mancia and others 2007)

List 2. Sub-Clinical Organ Damage (OD)

Other risk factors, OD or disease	Blood pressure levels (grades according the ESC/ESH Classification) in mmHg				
	SBP 120-129 or DBP 80-84 (Normal)	**SBP 130-139 or DBP 85-89** (High normal)	**SBP 140-159 or DBP 90-99** (Grade 1HT)	**SBP 160-179 or DBP 100-109** (Grade 2 HT)	**SBP≥180 or DBP ≥110** (Grade 3 HT)
No other risk factors	No	No	Low	Moderate	High
1-2 risk factors	Low	Low	Moderate	Moderate	Very High
3 or more risk factors, MS, OD or Diabetes	Moderate	High	High	High	Very High
Established CV or renal disease	Very High	Very High	Very High	Very High	Very High

*Adapted from "2007 ESC/ESH Recommendations" (Mancia and others 2007)
Notes and legends: SBP: systolic blood pressure; DBP: diastolic blood pressure; CV: cardiovascular; HT: hypertension. Low, moderate, high and very high risk refer to 10 year risk of a CV fatal or non-fatal event. The term 'added' indicates that in all categories risk is greater than average.
OD: subclinical organ damage; MS: metabolic syndrome.

Table 4. Stratification of Cardiovascular Risk expressed as added cardiovascular risk

4.3 Hypertension management strategies

The treatment of hypertension itself is based on prevention measures (World Hypertension League 1992), non-pharmacological measures (Cooper and others 1998) and a pharmacological treatment (Dominguez and others 2006). Table 5 shows the advocated (Mancia and others 2007) therapeutic approach based on cardiovascular risk stratification as shown in **Table 4.**

Preventive strategies

Because of restrained economic conditions in the developing world, the greatest gains in controlling the Cardiovascular diseases epidemic lie in its prevention. In addition to prevention, awareness of having hypertensive is important. Efforts should be made to early detect hypertensive patients before irreversible organ damage, and to provide them with the best possible and affordable non-pharmacological and pharmacological treatment.

The preventive actions concern habits and lifestyle monitoring. Those include the important but relatively low cost preventive measures: reduction in dietary salt intake (Douglas and others 2003), and a greater awareness of the implications of obesity (Bovet and others 2002). There is good evidence that a reduction in salt intake reduces blood pressure and that black people are more sensitive than white people in this regard (Cappuccio and others 2000). Other measures as increased exercise (Opie and Seedat 2005), stopping smoking (Ambrose and Barua 2004) and limiting alcohol intake (Appel and others 2003) are all attainable and can help in control of the hypertension as well.

Other risk factors, OD or disease	**Blood pressure (grades according the ESC/ESH Classification) in mmHg**				
	SBP 120-129 or DBP 80-84 (Normal)	**SBP 130-139 or DBP 85-89** (High normal)	**SBP 140-159 or DBP 90-99** (Grade 1HT)	**SBP 160-179 or DBP 100-109** (Grade 2 HT)	**SBP≥180 or DBP ≥110** (Grade 3 HT)
No other risk factors	No BP Intervention	No BP intervention	Lifestyle changes (several months) then drug treatment if BP uncontrolled	Lifestyle changes (several months) then drug treatment if BP uncontrolled	Lifestyle changes + Immediate drug treatment
1-2 risk factors	Lifestyle changes	Lifestyle changes	Lifestyle changes (several months) then drug treatment if BP uncontrolled	Lifestyle changes (several months) then drug treatment if BP uncontrolled	Lifestyle changes + Immediate drug treatment
3 or more risk factors, MS or OD	Lifestyle changes	Lifestyle changes + Consider drug treatment	Lifestyle changes + Drug treatment	Lifestyle changes + Drug treatment	Lifestyle changes + Immediate drug treatment
Diabetes	Lifestyle changes	Lifestyle changes + Drug treatment			
Established CV or renal disease	Lifestyle changes + Immediate drug treatment	Lifestyle changes + Immediate drug treatment	Lifestyle changes + Immediate drug treatment	Lifestyle changes + Immediate drug treatment	Lifestyle changes + Immediate drug treatment

Notes and legends: SBP: systolic blood pressure; DBP: diastolic blood pressure; CV: cardiovascular; HT: hypertension. OD: subclinical organ damage; MS: metabolic syndrome.

Table 5. Therapeutic approach for hypertension in adults [Adapted from 2007 ESC/ESH Recommendations] (Mancia and others 2007)

Diet control in developing countries remains a great challenge. The diet is highly linked to the population culture, to the food conservation, cooking, and other existing infrastructures. Salt reduction measures may be difficult in population using it for food conservation. The restructured diets like promoted in Dietary Approaches to Stop Hypertension (DASH) (Sacks and others 1999; Svetkey and others 1999), may not apply to other low resource settings because those measures require structures of preparation, conservation and other infrastructures and resources which are not available. Therefore, preventive measures must be based on available food locally, and take into account the food and cooking habits of the population. All lifestyle modifications must emphasize the role of regular physical activity.

Another important measure to promote is the regular check of blood pressure for all (also young) adult people, in contrast to western countries where this measure is taken above a certain age.

Pharmacological treatment

The pharmacological treatment of hypertension includes several classes of anti-hypertensive drugs (Brewster and others 2004). The 5 main classes with proven effect on hard endpoints are [1] beta-blockers (BB), [2] diuretics (DIU), [3] calcium channel blockers (CCB), [4] angiotensin converting enzyme inhibitors (ACEI) and [5] angiotensin receptor blockers (ARB). Additional classes also used are centrally acting drugs, peripheral sympatholytics and direct vasodilators. The WHO recommends only four drug classes (BB, DIU, CCB and ACEI) from the five first-line classes on its essential drug list (World Health Organization 2007).

Most surveys evaluating the prescribing behaviours of practising physicians revealed that monotherapy is less preferred (one third of cases) versus polypharmacy (Anthierens and others 2010; O'Riordan and others 2008; Pittrow and others 2004). In monotherapy, beta-blockers have been found the drugs of choice prescribed at the level of primary health care centres in many places. Among the various beta-blockers that are approved worldwide for the treatment of hypertension, cardioselective beta-blockers atenolol and metoprolol and the non-selective beta-blocker propranolol are the commonly used. Although advocated by current guidelines, the diuretics are the not often given. In the Polypharmacy group, of combinations given as first-line nearly always include diuretics. They are combined with CCBs or ACEIs or other diuretics.

Overall the prescribers behaviour is far from homogenous, and the existence of international guidelines may not help a lot, if they are not adapted to local or specific situations.

First-line drugs in hypertension

As far as the first-line drug in treatment of hypertension is concerned, the opening debate may be the choice between monotherapy versus combination therapy as first line for the treatment of uncomplicated arterial hypertension. However, this debate seems less supported as it may be more cost-effective to start with a single drug and try to control the blood pressure combined with non-pharmacological treatment.

Historically the selection of the first-line drug remains debatable (Lindholm and others 2005). Since 1993 WHO/ISH guidelines sub-committee recommended that diuretics, beta-blockers, ACE inhibitors, calcium channel blockers and alpha-blockers are first-line drugs suitable for treatment of patients with hypertension. This view was again endorsed by the guidelines subcommittee of WHO/ISH in 1999 with the addition of a new class of antihypertensive, angiotensin II receptor antagonists. The United States JNC VI (Johnson

2008)in May 2003 and British Hypertension Society guidelines(Johnson 2008) both recommended low-dose diuretics and beta-blockers as first-line treatment unless there are compelling contraindications or compelling indications for other drug classes. These differences are of considerable importance, because pharmaceutical companies are inevitably keen to promote the more liberal international (WHO/ISH) guidelines even in countries with national guidelines that recommend a different policy (Ho and others 2010; Johnson 2008).

The aim of this section will not be to prolong the debate but to extract a clear message and recommendations from existing information.

To suggest any other first-line drug, it is important to focus on comparative analyses of cardiovascular outcomes, efficacy in reducing blood pressure (BP), adverse effects, contra-indications and cost.

What then should be our final choice for routine first-line antihypertensive treatment? Some patients have compelling indications or contraindications for one drug class or another, but the vast majority do not. For these patients the trial evidence would not support the use of selective alpha-blockers or calcium channel blockers as routine first-line treatment (Jackson and Ramsay 2002). The evidence would justify the use of low-dose diuretics, beta-blockers, or ACE inhibitors as routine first-line treatment, with nothing important to choose between them. When there is really nothing to choose between drugs, it is self-evident that the cheapest drug should be preferred. In most health care systems, that will be a low dose of a thiazide diuretic (Jackson and Ramsay 2002).

Coming back to low resource settings, evidences support the use of thiazide diuretics as first line and in monotherapy as well, followed if uncontrolled blood pressure by association with a very small dose of Reserpine where the affordability is very low (Twagirumukiza and Van Bortel 2011). In places where the treatment affordability is optimum, the diuretics can be associated to CCBs or ACEIs or other diuretics (Twagirumukiza and Van Bortel 2011), or to BBs in situations where their efficacy has been documented and approved (Fig.1).

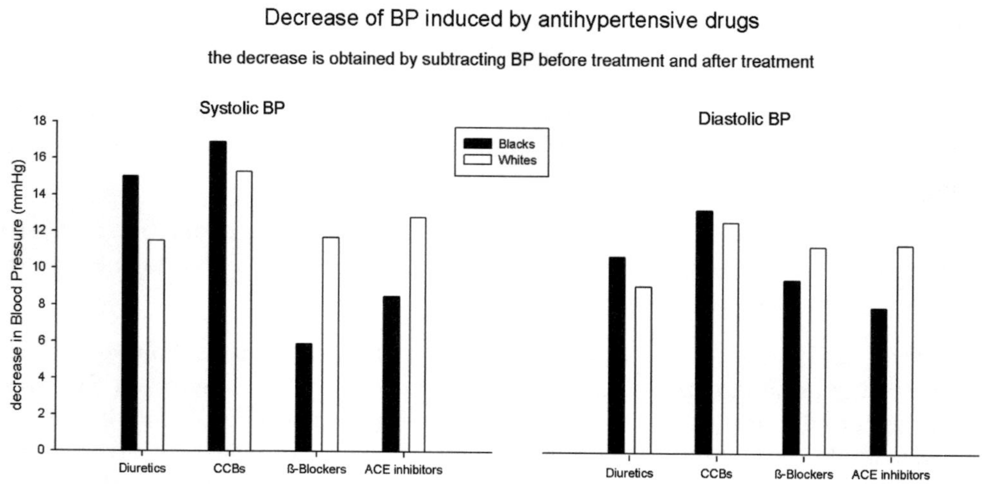

CCBs: calcium channel blockers; **BP**: blood pressure.

Fig. 1. Decrease in BP with antihypertensive drug treatments in Black/Whites [adapted from Brewster et al(Brewster and others 2004)]

4.4 The use of guidelines: Applicable for all?

There are 3 main international guidelines suggested for the management of hypertension in the world : (1) the 2003 WHO/ISH Statement on Management of Hypertension(Whitworth 2003); (2) the European guideline, issued by European Society of Hypertension (ESH) and European society of cardiology (ESC): the 2007 ESH/ESC guidelines (Mancia and others 2007) and (3) the United States of America (US) guideline, issued by the Joint National Committee on Prevention, Detection, Evaluation, and Treatment of High Blood Pressure: the 2003 JNC-7 report (Chobanian and others 2003). Besides those main guidelines others documents and reports have been published to help in management of hypertension in particular settings, including: (1) the consensus statement of the Hypertension in African-Americans working group of the International Society on Hypertension in Blacks (Douglas and others 2003), and (2) the 2002 WHO Cardiovascular Risk Management Package in Low- and Medium-Resource Settings (World Health Organization (WHO) 2002).

However, those international guidelines may not be applicable in all low resources settings as specificities can exist in the concerned population. For instance the content of non-pharmacological treatment that is mainly based on lifestyle change and promoted by a patient education package remains similar in western developed countries and developing countries. Nevertheless, a difference in outcomes can be expected from the high illiteracy rate in developing countries that may require different educational methods. Moreover, the population cultures and the real way of living (activities, historic habits like salt intake, etc) must be taken into account.

This chapter will provide a suggested algorithm for management of hypertension from the community level and with emphasis on the primary health care setting and public health perspective.

Whatever guideline considered, we cannot assume its applicability to all regions, even if they have been drafted on regional basis. For instance, the limited resources devoted toward health care in many developing countries limit the number of health facilities and existence of health insurance schemes (Ndiaye and others 2007). In this setting, cases of malignant hypertension, with target organ damage are frequent (Mensah and others 1994). Pooled data from inhospital studies published between 1998 and 2008, show that the most frequent complication reported downward are heart failure, renal failure, stroke and coronary heart disease (CHD) (Twagirumukiza and Van Bortel 2011).

Additionally, although the benefit of treatment is established(Brewster and others 2004), the treatment cost and accessibility must be more emphasized in developing countries (Twagirumukiza and others 2010).

Also, ethnic differences have been described also in drug response(Johnson 2008) in Caucasians versus blacks, but since there is limited clinical trial data from the African region, it is not fully clear whether the differences observed in USA can be fully extrapolated to African or other ethnic groups. Nevertheless, the available data from studies conducted in sub-Saharan Africa, confirm notable differences in response to β-blockers (Preston and others 1998), ACE inhibitors (Sareli and others 2001), and angiotensin receptor blockers (Wright, Jr. and others 2005), and stress the efficacy of diuretics, particularly thiazides (Wright, Jr. and others 2008). A meta-analysis, published in 2004 (Brewster and others 2004), evaluating 15 clinical trials published between 1984 and 1998 reported differences in antihypertensive response between blacks and whites of comparable groups, highlights the fact that whites tend to respond to all the drug classes (Figure 1) whereas blacks generally respond better than whites to diuretics and calcium channel blockers, and whites respond better than blacks to ACE inhibitors and β-blockers (Opie and Seedat 2005).

In many developing countries, two other aspects must be added in all hypertension treatment strategies: the quality of the drug and its price, which influence the efficacy of the treatment, its accessibility and adherence. Contrary to western countries where the drugs registration process and other related regulations are meticulous, in sub-Saharan Africa the quality of drug is not checked at entrance (Caudron and others 2008), the drug market is not fully controlled (Andriollo O and others 1998), registration processes are very often lacking (Caudron and others 2008) and the pharmacovigilance systems are not yet established everywhere. Moreover, the storage in tropical conditions with high humidity and high temperature deteriorate the drugs potency and/or bioavailability (Twagirumukiza and others 2009a).

The big contrast between western and sub-Saharan Africa settings in this area is the affordability to the treatment. In sub-Saharan Africa the price of the majority of antihypertensive drugs is higher than indicated in the International Drugs Prices Indicator Guide (IDPIG) (Management Sciences for Health (MSH) and World Health Organization (WHO) 2007), and treatments with an antihypertensive drug are in general cheaper when the drug is on the National Essential Medicine List (NEML). Drug price monitoring in every country, putting drugs on NEML, and setting up regulations on the drug market, are the main actions to reduce and/or stabilize the prices of drugs (Health Action International 2008) and to improve the affordability and accessibility to the hypertension treatment.

4.5 Public health perspective

Based on available data and the 2002 WHO Cardiovascular Risk Management Package in Low- and Medium-Resource Settings(World Health Organization (WHO) 2002), a set of algorithms have been proposed (Twagirumukiza and Van Bortel 2011) for hypertension management in low resources settings and particularly in sub-Saharan Africa. The following 2 algorithms (Figure 2 &3) are extracted from the full set of them. Since every region has its own disparities between countries, those algorithm have flexibility to be adapted according to the country situation and it involves the use of total cardiovascular risk assessment, based on WHO cardiovascular risk assessment charts (Mendis and others 2007).

The entry point is the suggestion of measuring blood pressure in all adults persons (25 years and above) at community level (commonly at the Community Health Worker/Advisor post)

The second step concerns those people detected with severe hypertension (sent immediately to the near health center) or those with hypertension grade 1 and 2 not responding to non-pharmacological treatment. Emphasis is to be made on the length of the follow up period on non-pharmacological treatment which is a maximum of 3 months for grade 2 hypertension and 6 months for the grade 1 hypertension.

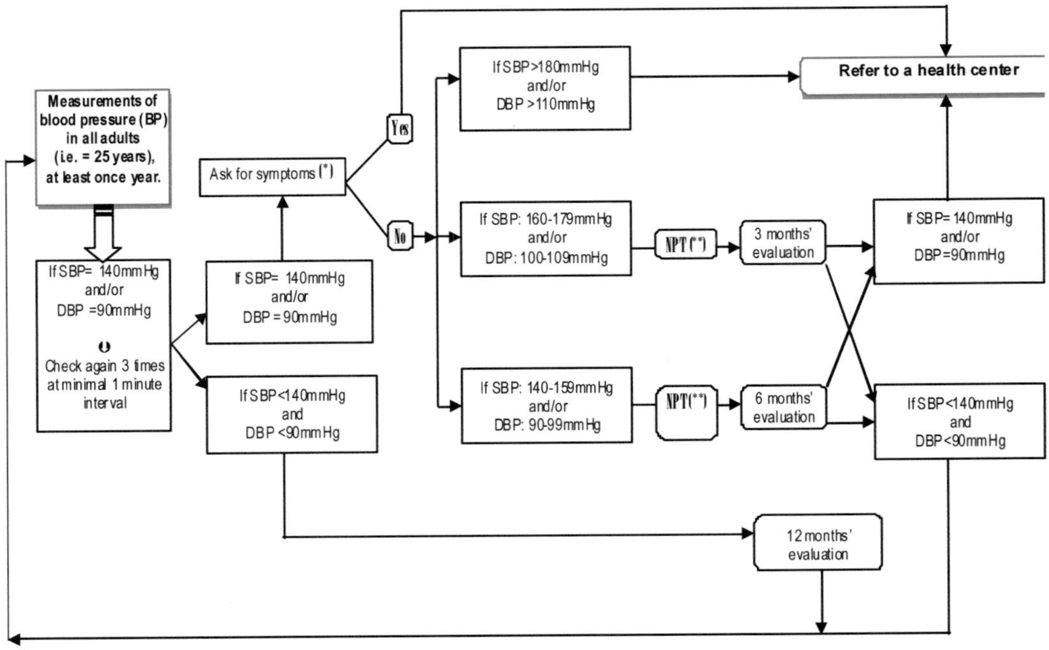

Legends: NPT: Non-pharmacological treatment; **SBP:** Systolic blood pressure; **DBP:** Diastolic blood pressure

Notes:(*) Symptoms to ask (Yes means the person answers yes at least to one of following questions):
- Shortness of breath on small exercise (like climbing a small distance, walking, etc)
- Both feet swollen.

(**)Non pharmacological treatment (NPT) includes:
- Stop smoking (keep in mind all kind of tobacco use)
- Overweight reduction and recommendation of a regular physical activity
- Dietetic measures: (Salt reduction, promote fresh fruits and vegetables intake, fatty food limitation, minimizing alcohol intake)

Fig. 2. Hypertension management strategy at the community level: At least, where a community health advisor/worker is available. (adapted from Twagirumukiza M et al, 2011)(Twagirumukiza and Van Bortel 2011)

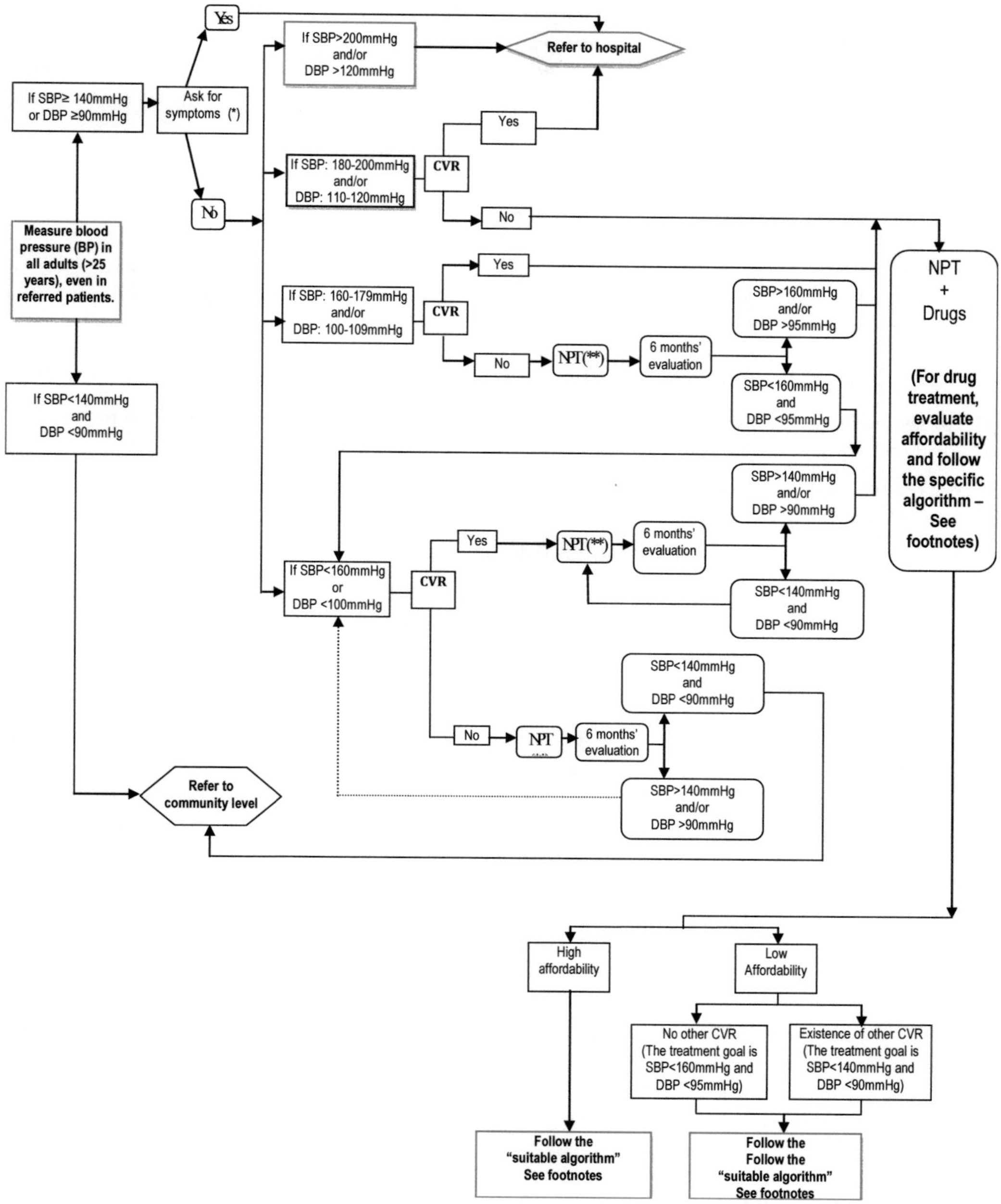

Legends: **ECG=** Electrocardiography; **NPT:** Non-pharmacological treatment; **CVR:** Cardiovascular risk factors; **SBP:** Systolic blood pressure; **DBP:** Diastolic blood pressure

Notes: [1] Minimal equipment: urine sticks for protein and glucose and preferentially a standard Electrocardiography.
[2] At CVR evaluation "Yes" means at least one cardiovascular risk factor is present; the cardiovascular factors to detect are:

a. Proteinuria (using dipsticks)
b. Glucosuria (using dipsticks). If positive follow also instructions for diabetes.

c. The left ventricular hypertrophy(LVH) on ECG; defined by a Cornell product parameter (positive if >2440 mm*msec). The parameter is calculated as follows:
   - Cornell product = (RaVL + SV3) × QRS duration (meaning the product of QRS duration with the sum of the R wave in lead "aVL" and the "S" wave in lead "V3"). The RaVL, SV3, QRS and V3 being ECG waves.
   - To measure QRS duration on ECG, recorded at a speed of 25 mm/sec:
   - Principles:
     - 1mV=10mm in the vertical direction.
     - Each small 1-mm square represents 0.04sec (40msec) in time and 0.1mV in voltage.
     - QRS duration: counting 1-mm square cell of the ECG, paper corresponding to the beginning and the end of QRS complex (horizontally), and then multiply the number by 40 msec.
   - R and S wave voltage are obtained by counting the number of 1-mm square cell (vertically) corresponding to the wave height (amplitude).

[3] The sentence "Follow the suitable algorithm- See footnotes" at the end of fig 3 refers to the algorithm which can be found in subsequent publication (not given here).

Whet it refers to the patient affordability, this can be evaluated based on patient-doctor communication but also to the socio-economic data provided in his medical record (file) and on patient interview.

[4] The (*) and (**) signs refer to the same legend as in figure 1.

Fig. 3. Hypertension management algorithm at the health centre: the first step (adapted from Twagirumukiza M et al, 2011)(Twagirumukiza and Van Bortel 2011)

4.6 Challenges and opportunities

Currently in many developing countries the global health initiatives and governments commitment to tackle the non-communicable diseases (De Maeseneer J. and others 2011) provide an optimistic development which will enhance the management of chronic diseases in general and hypertension in particular.

The health care systems are constantly improving as the primary health care (PHC) programs are starting in various regions (De Maeseneer J 2009). Certainly the Primary Health Care (PHC)-in line with recommendations of the World Health Report 2008 (De Maeseneer J 2009), may play an important role in implementation of all chronic disease treatment strategies. Nowadays international partners put valuable efforts into training of family physicians in developing and particularly in African countries (De Maeseneer J 2009). Most of those family physicians are working in the district health hospital. However, in the future, they are intended to be located in primary health care centers and when a primary health care centre has a family physician, the management algorithm should be adapted, as referral to the hospital will be less needed.

About the drug quality (Twagirumukiza and others 2009a) and drug market regulations, it is important to mention that during recent years, there have been efforts to strengthen regulatory systems and the World Health Organization (WHO) has comprehensively assessed more than 20 regulatory authorities in sub-Saharan Africa and in Latina America, south Asia and other developing regions. WHO and others initiatives have trained a number of regulatory officials to strengthen and harmonize the drugs regulatory processes. Even if it's a long way to go to have national regulators and pharmacovigilance centres fully operational in sub-Saharan Africa countries, things have started moving in the right direction. WHO and international donors have also increasingly invested both in monitoring the quality of products and in building up functional quality control laboratories through the WHO respective prequalification program.

Finally, the important cross-cutting and global issues should be considered in all thinking stages of setting up the treatment of hypertension: people centred care, continuity of health care, adherence to treatment, drug interactions, contra-indications and comorbidities, and the essential broad debate of equity in health care.

5. Conclusions

Although it is important to consider the current knowledge of medicine for the treatment of hypertension, particular consideration should be given to cost-effectiveness and affordability of antihypertensive medicines in primary health care settings of the developing countries. This consideration is justified because many low and middle income countries have severe resource constraints and available resources currently do not allow to treat all patients according to some international guidelines. Therefore, strategies have to be developed to maximally reduce risk for and from hypertension within the limited budget. Such strategy should take into account many local socio-economic and demographic particularities. The hypertension management strategy must be based on patient's cardiovascular risk and not only on his blood pressure level. Additionally the common sense says that for the same result and efficacy the cheapest is the best choice. Therefore it's obvious that the drug prices and quality details must constitute an added criterion when choosing an antihypertensive agent. Developing countries should be encouraged to establish a list with medicine prices using the real patient price, and this list has to be updated at least every year, and the prescribers should be encouraged to choose the cheapest between the available drugs which fulfil the quality criteria.

Beyond that, the management of hypertension in primary health care settings suppose a complete rebuild of health care systems and empowering of the community. The detection and monitoring should be done at community levels and early treatment at primary health care level. As already repeated by many authors, the efforts to effectively improve the control of hypertension should be based on a patient-centred care concept, rather than disease centred care. This suppose a thorough understanding of the characteristics of patients, the dynamics of the health care system and, most importantly, on the work and function of the primary care physician as the gatekeeper.

6. References

[1] Ambrose JA, Barua RS. 2004. The pathophysiology of cigarette smoking and cardiovascular disease: an update. J Am Coll Cardiol 43(10):1731-7.

[2] Andriollo O, Machuron L, Videau JY, Abelli C, Plot S, Muller D. 1998. Supplies for humanitarian aid and development countries: The quality of essential multisources drugs. Sciences et Techniques Pharmaceutiques (STP Pharma Pratiques) 8(2):137-55.

[3] Anthierens S, Tansens A, Petrovic M, Christiaens T. 2010. Qualitative insights into general practitioners views on polypharmacy. BMC Fam Pract 11:65.

[4] Appel LJ, Champagne CM, Harsha DW, Cooper LS, Obarzanek E, Elmer PJ, Stevens VJ, Vollmer WM, Lin PH, Svetkey LP, Stedman SW, Young DR. 2003. Effects of

comprehensive lifestyle modification on blood pressure control: Main results of the PREMIER clinical trial. Journal of the American Medical Association 289(16):2083-93.

[5] Birkett NJ. 1997. The effect of alternative criteria for hypertension on estimates of prevalence and control. J Hypertens 15(3):237-44.

[6] Bovet P, Ross AG, Gervasoni JP, Mkamba M, Mtasiwa DM, Lengeler C, Whiting D, Paccaud F. 2002. Distribution of blood pressure, body mass index and smoking habits in the urban population of Dar es Salaam, Tanzania, and associations with socioeconomic status. International Journal of Epidemiology 31(1):240-7.

[7] Brewster LM, Van Montfrans GA, Kleijnen J. 2004. Systematic review: Antihypertensive drug therapy in black patients. Annals of Internal Medicine 141(8):614-27.

[8] Cappuccio FP, Plange-Rhule J, Phillips RO, Eastwood JB. 2000. Prevention of hypertension and stroke in Africa. Lancet 356(9230):677-8.

[9] Caudron JM, Ford N, Henkens M, Mace C, Kiddle-Monroe R, Pinel J. 2008. Substandard medicines in resource-poor settings: a problem that can no longer be ignored. Tropical Medicine and International Health 13(8):1062-72.

[10] Chalmers J, MacMahon S, Mancia G, Whitworth J, Beilin L, Hansson L, Neal B, Rodgers A, Ni MC, Clark T. 1999. 1999 World Health Organization-International Society of Hypertension Guidelines for the management of hypertension. Guidelines sub-committee of the World Health Organization. Clin Exp Hypertens 21(5-6):1009-60.

[11] Chemla D. 2006. Factors which may influence mean arterial pressure measurement. Can J Anaesth 53(4):421-2.

[12] Chobanian AV, Bakris GL, Black HR, Cushman WC, Green LA, Izzo JL, Jr., Jones DW, Materson BJ, Oparil S, Wright JT, Jr., Roccella EJ. 2003. The Seventh Report of the Joint National Committee on Prevention, Detection, Evaluation, and Treatment of High Blood Pressure: the JNC 7 report. Journal of the American Medical Association 289(19):2560-72.

[13] Christiaens T. 2008. Cardiovascular risk tables. BMJ 336(7659):1445-6.

[14] Cooper RS, Rotimi CN, Kaufman JS, Muna WF, Mensah GA. 1998. Hypertension treatment and control in sub-Saharan Africa: The epidemiological basis for policy. British Medical Journal 316(7131):614-7.

[15] De Maeseneer J. 2009. Primary Health Care in Africa: Now more then ever! Afr J Prm Health Care Fam Med 1(1):112-5.

[16] De Maeseneer J., Roberts RG, Demarzo M, Heath I, Sewankambo N, Kidd MR, van WC, Egilman D, Boelen C, Willems S. 2011. Tackling NCDs: a different approach is needed. Lancet.

[17] Dominguez LJ, Galioto A, Ferlisi A, Pineo A, Putignano E, Belvedere M, Costanza G, Barbagallo M. 2006. Ageing, lifestyle modifications, and cardiovascular disease in developing countries. Journal of Nutrition, Health & Aging 10(2):143-9.

[18] Douglas JG, Bakris GL, Epstein M, Ferdinand KC, Ferrario C, Flack JM, Jamerson KA, Jones WE, Haywood LJ, Maxey R, Ofili EO, Saunders E, Schiffrin EL, Sica DA, Sowers JR, Vidt DG. 2003. Management of high blood pressure in African Americans: consensus statement of the Hypertension in African Americans Working Group of the International Society on Hypertension in Blacks. Archives of Internal Medicine 163(5):525-41.

[19] Fields LE, Burt VL, Cutler JA, Hughes J, Roccella EJ, Sorlie P. 2004. The burden of adult hypertension in the United States 1999 to 2000: a rising tide. Hypertension 44(4):398-404.

[20] Gaziano TA. 2005. Cardiovascular disease in the developing world and its cost-effective management. Circulation 112(23):3547-53.

[21] Health Action International, HAI. Monitoring medicine prices, availability and affordability : pilot countries' reports. HAI 2008;Available from: URL: http://www.haiweb.org/medicineprices/. Accessed on: December 20, 2011

[22] Ho PM, Zeng C, Tavel HM, Selby JV, O'Connor PJ, Margolis KL, Magid DJ. 2010. Trends in first-line therapy for hypertension in the Cardiovascular Research Network Hypertension Registry, 2002-2007. Arch Intern Med 170(10):912-3.

[23] Jackson PR, Ramsay LE. 2002. First-line treatment for hypertension. Eur Heart J 23(3):179-82.

[24] Jha P, Chaloupka F. 1999. Tobacco control in developing countries. On behalf of The Human Development Network, the World Bank, and the Economics Advisory Service, World Health Organization. New York: Oxford University Press.

[25] John KJ Li. 2000. The arterial circulation : physical principals and clinical application. Piscataway, New Jersey, USA: Humana Press. 1 p.

[26] Johnson JA. 2008. Ethnic differences in cardiovascular drug response: Potential contribution of pharmacogenetics. Circulation 118(13):1383-93.

[27] Kearney PM, Whelton M, Reynolds K, Muntner P, Whelton PK, He J. 2005. Global burden of hypertension: analysis of worldwide data. Lancet 365(9455):217-23.

[28] Khosla N, Black HR. 2006. Expanding the definition of hypertension to incorporate global cardiovascular risk. Curr Hypertens Rep 8(5):384-90.

[29] Lawes CM, Vander HS, Rodgers A. 2008. Global burden of blood-pressure-related disease, 2001. Lancet 371(9623):1513-8.

[30] Lindholm LH, Carlberg B, Samuelsson O. 2005. Should beta blockers remain first choice in the treatment of primary hypertension? A meta-analysis. Lancet 366(9496):1545-53.

[31] Lopez AD, Mathers CD, Ezzati M, Jamison DT, Murray CJ. 2006. Global and regional burden of disease and risk factors, 2001: systematic analysis of population health data. Lancet 367(9524):1747-57.

[32] MacDonald TM, Morant SV. 2008. Prevalence and treatment of isolated and concurrent hypertension and hypercholesterolaemia in the United Kingdom. Br J Clin Pharmacol 65(5):775-86.

[33] Management Sciences for Health (MSH), World Health Organization (WHO). 2007. International drug price indicator guide 2007. 2007 ed. MSH, WHO. 1 p.

[34] Mancia G, de BG, Dominiczak A, Cifkova R, Fagard RH, Germano G, Grassi G, Heagerty AM, Kjeldsen SE, Laurent S, Narkiewicz K, Ruilope L, Rynkiewicz A, Schmieder RE, Boudier HA, Zanchetti A, Vahanian A, Camm J, De CR, Dean V, Dickstein K, Filippatos G, Funck-Brentano C, Hellemans I, Kristensen SD, McGregor K, Sechtem U, Silber S, Tendera M, Widimsky P, Zamorano JL, Erdine S, Kiowski W, Gabiti-Rosei E, Ambrosioni E, Lindholm LH, Viigimaa M, Adamopoulos S, Gabiti-Rosei E, Ambrosioni E, Bertomeu V, Clement D, Erdine S, Farsang C, Gaita D, Lip GY, Mallion JM, Manolis AJ, Nilsson PM, O'Brien E, Ponikowski P, Redon J, Ruschitzka F, Tamargo J, Van Zwieten P, Waeber B,

Williams B. 2007. 2007 Guidelines for the Management of Arterial Hypertension: The Task Force for the Management of Arterial Hypertension of the European Society of Hypertension (ESH) and of the European Society of Cardiology (ESC). Journal of Hypertension 25(6):1105-87.
[35] Mendis S, Lindholm LH, Mancia G, Whitworth J, Alderman M, Lim S, Heagerty T. 2007. World Health Organization (WHO) and International Society of Hypertension (ISH) risk prediction charts: assessment of cardiovascular risk for prevention and control of cardiovascular disease in low and middle-income countries. J Hypertens 25(8):1578-82.
[36] Mensah GA. 2003. A heart-healthy and "stroke-free" world through policy development, systems change, and environmental supports: a 2020 vision for sub-Saharan Africa. Ethn Dis 13(2 Suppl 2):S4-12.
[37] Mensah GA, Barkey NL, Cooper RS. 1994. Spectrum of hypertensive target organ damage in Africa: a review of published studies. Journal of Human Hypertension 8(11):799-808.
[38] Mufunda J, Rufaro Chatora, Yustina Ndambakuwa, Peter Nyarango ea. 2006. Emerging Non-Communicable Disease Epidemic in Africa: Preventive Measures from the WHO Regional Office for Africa. Ethn Dis 16(2):521-6.
[39] Murray CJ, Lopez AD. 1997. Mortality by cause for eight regions of the world: Global Burden of Disease Study. Lancet 349(9061):1269-76.
[40] Ndiaye P, Soors W, Criel B. 2007. Editorial: a view from beneath: Community health insurance in Africa. Tropical Medicine and International Health 12(2):157-61.
[41] Nichols WW., O'Rourke MF., Vlachopoulos C. 2011. McDonald's Blood Flow in Arteries: Theoretical, Experimental and Clinical Principles. Oxford Univ Pr.
[42] O'Riordan S, Mackson J, Weekes L. 2008. Self-reported prescribing for hypertension in general practice. J Clin Pharm Ther 33(5):483-8.
[43] Opie LH, Seedat YK. 2005. Hypertension in sub-Saharan African populations. Circulation 112(23):3562-8.
[44] Papadopoulos DP, Makris TK. 2007. Masked hypertension definition, impact, outcomes: a critical review. J Clin Hypertens (Greenwich) 9(12):956-63.
[45] Pestana JA, Steyn K, Leiman A, Hartzenberg GM. 1996. The direct and indirect costs of cardiovascular disease in South Africa in 1991. South African Medical Journal 86(6):679-84.
[46] Pittrow D, Kirch W, Bramlage P, Lehnert H, Hofler M, Unger T, Sharma AM, Wittchen HU. 2004. Patterns of antihypertensive drug utilization in primary care. Eur J Clin Pharmacol 60(2):135-42.
[47] Preston RA, Materson BJ, Reda DJ, Williams DW, Hamburger RJ, Cushman WC, Anderson RJ. 1998. Age-race subgroup compared with renin profile as predictors of blood pressure response to antihypertensive therapy. Department of Veterans Affairs Cooperative Study Group on Antihypertensive Agents. Journal of the American Medical Association 280(13):1168-72.
[48] Reddy KS, Yusuf S. 1998. Emerging epidemic of cardiovascular disease in developing countries. Circulation 97(6):596-601.
[49] Roger VL., Go AS., Lloyd-Jones DM., Adams RJ, Berry JD, Brown TM, Carnethon MR, Dai S, de SG, Ford ES, Fox CS, Fullerton HJ, Gillespie C, Greenlund KJ, Hailpern SM, Heit JA, Ho PM, Howard VJ, Kissela BM, Kittner SJ, Lackland DT, Lichtman

JH, Lisabeth LD, Makuc DM, Marcus GM, Marelli A, Matchar DB, McDermott MM, Meigs JB, Moy CS, Mozaffarian D, Mussolino ME, Nichol G, Paynter NP, Rosamond WD, Sorlie PD, Stafford RS, Turan TN, Turner MB, Wong ND, Wylie-Rosett J. 2011. Heart disease and stroke statistics-2011 update: a report from the American Heart Association. Circulation 123(4):e18-e209.

[50] Sacks FM, Appel LJ, Moore TJ, Obarzanek E, Vollmer WM, Svetkey LP, Bray GA, Vogt TM, Cutler JA, Windhauser MM, Lin PH, Karanja N. 1999. A dietary approach to prevent hypertension: a review of the Dietary Approaches to Stop Hypertension (DASH) Study. Clinical Cardiology 22(7 Suppl):III6-10.

[51] Sareli P, Radevski IV, Valtchanova ZP, Libhaber E, Candy GP, Den HE, Libhaber C, Skudicky D, Wang JG, Staessen JA. 2001. Efficacy of different drug classes used to initiate antihypertensive treatment in black subjects: results of a randomized trial in Johannesburg, South Africa. Archives of Internal Medicine 161(7):965-71.

[52] Svetkey LP, Sacks FM, Obarzanek E, Vollmer WM, Appel LJ, Lin PH, Karanja NM, Harsha DW, Bray GA, Aickin M, Proschan MA, Windhauser MM, Swain JF, McCarron PB, Rhodes DG, Laws RL. 1999. The DASH Diet, Sodium Intake and Blood Pressure Trial (DASH-sodium): rationale and design. DASH-Sodium Collaborative Research Group. Journal of American Dietetic Association 99(8 Suppl):S96-104.

[53] Twagirumukiza M, Annemans L, Kips JG, Bienvenu E, Van Bortel LM. 2010. Prices of antihypertensive medicines in sub-Saharan Africa and alignment to WHO's model list of essential medicines. Trop Med Int Health 15(3):350-61.

[54] Twagirumukiza M, Cosijns A, Pringels E, Remon JP, Vervaet C, Van BL. 2009a. Influence of tropical climate conditions on the quality of antihypertensive drugs from Rwandan pharmacies. Am J Trop Med Hyg 81(5):776-81.

[55] Twagirumukiza M, De Bacquer D, Kips J, vander Stichele R, De Backer G, Van Bortel LM. 2009b. Hypertension in sub-Saharan Africa (SSA): Low Prevalence, But High Risk. J Hypertens 27:S410.

[56] Twagirumukiza M, De BD, Kips JG, de BG, Stichele RV, Van Bortel LM. 2011. Current and projected prevalence of arterial hypertension in sub-Saharan Africa by sex, age and habitat: an estimate from population studies. J Hypertens 29(7):1243-52.

[57] Twagirumukiza M, Van Bortel LM. 2011. Management of hypertension at the community level in sub-Saharan Africa (SSA): towards a rational use of available resources. J Hum Hypertens 25(1):47-56.

[58] Unwin N, Setel P, Rashid S, Mugusi F, Mbanya JC, Kitange H, Hayes L, Edwards R, Aspray T, Alberti KG. 2001. Noncommunicable diseases in sub-Saharan Africa: Where do they feature in the health research agenda? Bulletin of the World Health Organization 79(10):947-53.

[59] Van Bortel LM, De BT, De BM. 2011. How to treat arterial stiffness beyond blood pressure lowering? J Hypertens 29(6):1051-3.

[60] Whitworth JA. 2003. 2003 World Health Organization (WHO)/International Society of Hypertension (ISH) statement on management of hypertension. Journal of Hypertension 21(11):1983-92.

[61] World Health Organization. 2007. The selection and use of essential medicines 2007. 15th Model list of essential medicines. WHO Technical Report Series(946):1-162.

[62] World Health Organization, J Mackay, G.Mensah. The Atlas of Heart Disease and Stroke, 2004. WHO. 1-112. 2004. Geneva, WHO.

[63] World Health Organization (WHO). 2002. CVD-Risk Management Package for Low and Medium Resource Settings. Geneva: WHO; 7 p. Available from.

[64] World Hypertension League. 1992. Can non-pharmacological interventions reduce doses of drugs needed for the treatment of hypertension? Bulletin of the World Health Organization 70(6):685-90.

[65] Wright JT, Jr., Dunn JK, Cutler JA, Davis BR, Cushman WC, Ford CE, Haywood LJ, Leenen FH, Margolis KL, Papademetriou V, Probstfield JL, Whelton PK, Habib GB. 2005. Outcomes in hypertensive black and nonblack patients treated with chlorthalidone, amlodipine, and lisinopril. Journal of the American Medical Association 293(13):1595-608.

[66] Wright JT, Jr., Harris-Haywood S, Pressel S, Barzilay J, Baimbridge C, Bareis CJ, Basile JN, Black HR, Dart R, Gupta AK, Hamilton BP, Einhorn PT, Haywood LJ, Jafri SZ, Louis GT, Whelton PK, Scott CL, Simmons DL, Stanford C, Davis BR. 2008. Clinical outcomes by race in hypertensive patients with and without the metabolic syndrome: Antihypertensive and Lipid-Lowering Treatment to Prevent Heart Attack Trial (ALLHAT). Archives of Internal Medicine 168(2):207-17.